THE HEALING WORD

The Healing Word

Preaching and Teaching Health Ministry

DEBORAH L. PATTERSON

THE PILGRIM PRESS
CLEVELAND

To those who minister
with healing words
in every place,

with thanks to the One
whose Word and Way
brings healing to all creation.

And a special word
of thanks
to my husband, Steve.

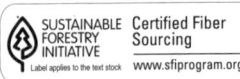

The Pilgrim Press, 700 Prospect Avenue, Cleveland, Ohio 44115
thepilgrimpress.com

© 2009 Deborah L. Patterson

Scripture quotations, unless otherwise noted, are from the New Revised Standard Version of the Bible, © 1989 by the Division of Christian Education of the National Council of Churches of Christ in the United States of America and are used by permission. Changes have been made for inclusivity.

All rights reserved. Published 2009

Printed in the United States of America on acid-free paper

13   12   11   10   09   5   4   3   2   1

Library of Congress Cataloging-in-Publication Data

Patterson, Deborah L., 1956–
    The healing word : preaching and teaching health ministry / Deborah L. Patterson.
      p. cm.
    Includes bibliographical references (p.   ).
    ISBN 978-0-8298-1849-9 (alk. paper)
    1. Medicine—Religious aspects—Christianity—Sermons. 2. Health—Religious aspects—Christianity—Sermons. 3. Parish nursing—Sermons. 4. Sermons, American—21st century. 5. Medicine—Religious aspects—Christianity—Meditations. 6. Health—Religious aspects—Christianity—Meditations. 7. Parish nursing—Meditations. I. Title.
BT732.P27 2009
261.5'61—dc22   2009003014

Contents

- Preface and Acknowledgments · vii

PART ONE: Called to Health Ministry · 1

SERMONS
1. Moved by Auto Rickshaw · 2
2. No Joy for You?! · 7

REFLECTIONS
3. Kidney Stones and Other Learning Experiences · 11
4. Mystics, Visionaries, and Healers · 13
5. Ministry Loves Company · 15
6. The Hidden Country Within · 16
- Discussion Questions · 18

PART TWO: Access to Health Care · 19

SERMONS
7. If Religion Was a Thing That Money Could Buy · 20
8. Rewriting Your Future · 28

REFLECTIONS
9. Praying for Health Care · 33
10. Health Care for an Arm and a Leg · 35
11. Downstairs on a First-Name Basis · 37
12. The Hardest Words · 39
- Discussion Questions · 41

PART THREE: Healthy Lifestyles · 43

SERMONS
13. Get My People Going!! · 44
14. And Their Eyes Were Opened · 48

REFLECTIONS
15. Finding Mayo · 53
16. Therefore, Choose Life · 55
17. Manna: When Enough Is Enough · 57
18. We Do Not Live by Stress Alone · 59
- Discussion Questions · 61

PART FOUR: Healthy Families · 63

SERMONS
19 · Suffer the Children · 64
20 · The Wisdom of Elders · 68

REFLECTIONS
21 · Lord, Help Us! · 72
22 · Identified: Flying Toilets · 78
23 · Getting Out of the House · 80
24 · No PAIN, No Gain · 82
· Discussion Questions · 84

PART FIVE: Healing Our Infirmities · 85

SERMONS
25 · Listening for the Sheer Silence · 86
26 · Good News for Lost Sheep · 90

REFLECTIONS
27 · Speaking of Death · 95
28 · Companions of Compassion · 97
29 · The Repentance That Leads to Life · 99
30 · The Underground Railroad of Compassion · 104
· Discussion Questions · 106

PART SIX: Health of Creation · 107

SERMONS
31 · Write the Vision; Make It Plain · 108
32 · The Earth Is Satisfied · 112

REFLECTIONS
33 · Where Has All the Oxygen Gone? · 115
34 · Praying for the Health of the World · 117
35 · Healing Christmas · 119
36 · God's Earth, Our Inheritance · 121
· Discussion Questions · 124
· Notes · 125
· Resources · 131
· Bibliography · 134

PREFACE and ACKNOWLEDGMENTS

*Jesus said, "I am the good shepherd;
I know my sheep and my sheep know me."*

John 10:14 NIV

Those of you of a "certain" age might remember watching a TV show called *To Tell the Truth*, on which the contestants tried to stump the celebrity guests about their identity. At the end of each round, the host Bud Collyer would ask, "Would the real [whoever] please stand up?"

Abraham Verghese, M.D., the senior associate chair for the Theory and Practice of Medicine at Stanford and a distinguished author, recently wrote of health care in the introduction to a collection of essays: "I think the patient in the bed has become a mere icon for the *real* patient, who is in the computer. The echocardiograms and CT scans and endoscopy images of the patient's innards, the numbers that describe the blood and organ functions, and, ergo, the real patient, is *in* the computer, visible to you with password and screen. The breathing, talking, anxious person in the bed, who wonders why the doctors appear so busy and yet so rarely come by, is an abstract entity." He goes on to say, "You might feel you are being pieced out: your heart to the *non-invasive* cardiologist, who might call in the *invasive* cardiologist if you need a cardiac catheterization, who, if you need angioplasty or a stent, gets the *interventional* cardiologist, who, if the root problem is a bad heart rhythm, calls in the cardiac *electrophysiologist*." He concludes by saying, "Reading these essays . . . is to hear a cry for a return to a simpler, more personal kind of medical care. *Talk to me!*"[1]

This collection of sermons, reflections, and questions for discussion offers an opportunity for clergy and parishioners, many of whom work in health care, and all of whom use health care from time to time, to talk to each other about issues facing communities today.

The recent survey of health ministries of Protestant churches done by the National Council of Churches of Christ in the USA found that congregations that had clergy who preached about health ministry were more likely to have health ministries.

Clergy typically feel ill-prepared to speak on the topic of health care. After all, few clergy are physicians, nurses, or health policy experts. Yet the church has been called to preach, teach, and heal, and clergy are leaders in the church. When we preach, people listen (we hope!). For heaven's sake, why else *would* we preach?

Few of us clergy are totally up-to-date on the wide range of health-care issues facing parishioners today—whether it be access to health care, optimal nutritional and exercise programs for promoting wellness, treatment options for the chronically or terminally ill, or the plethora of resources (and reimbursement options) for those needing additional assistance. But we *do* know that in 2008, more than forty-seven million people were uninsured in America, despite the United Nations' Declaration of Human Rights, which includes access to health care as a basic human right. We *do* know that there are many families who deal with mental illness or disabilities every day, for we see them in our congregations and communities. We *do* know that we live in a mobile society, where adult children often live far from their aging parents and worry about their increasing fragility, for we are called to assist them regularly. We *do* know that the church is called to follow Christ, one who healed all those who came to him, and who told us to go and do likewise. Healing ministry must be front and center in the church, as it was for Jesus. We have to talk about and practice health and wholeness, not just schedule health screenings, as we "talk the talk, and walk the walk."

The twelve sermons and twenty-four reflections or "discussion starters" that follow are divided up into six parts:

CALLED TO HEALTH MINISTRY
ACCESS TO HEALTH CARE
HEALTHY LIFESTYLES
HEALTHY FAMILIES
HEALING OUR INFIRMITIES
HEALTH OF CREATION

Each can be used as ideas for sermon topics or starters for adult education classes. The questions that follow each part can be used in preparation for writing one's sermons or to facilitate group discussion. This format would allow either for six weeks of sermons and adult education classes on health-related topics or for picking and choosing material as "food for thought" at any time during the course of a church year.

Several of these sermons were delivered in congregations and chapels in various settings. Chapter 21, ("Lord, Help Us!") on ministry to families with mental health issues, is adapted from material recently published in *The Clergy Journal*, and I am deeply indebted to its editor, Rebecca Grothe, for permission to use it here. A number of the "Reflections" grew out of meditations that first appeared in *Parish Nurse Perspectives*, a publication of the International Parish Nurse Resource Center for which I serve as editor. I take full responsibility for any errors that may appear in these pages.

To the outstanding staff of The Pilgrim Press, I give my deepest thanks, particularly to Kim M. Sadler, editorial director and Janice Brown, production director. It is indeed an honor to have a book published by the oldest surviving press in America. I am grateful for their interest in parish nursing and other health ministries. I am also indebted to Dr. Allen Mueller, former director of the Luhr Library at Eden Theological Seminary, for his help with citations, to Ulrike Guthrie for her thoughtful editing, to Kris Firth for her amazing commitment to editorial detail in shepherding this manuscript into its final form, to Rick Porter for a design that integrates form and function so well, and to the sharp eyes of proofreader, Dan Duffee.

Thank you also to the Health Task Force of the National Council of Churches, with representatives from many denominations working to bring together the efforts of health ministries across the land and abroad, whose vision and leadership help to provide direction for combined efforts in ministry.

Thank you to the Deaconess Foundation, whose leadership in supporting parish nursing is unparalleled, along with their groundbreaking work in improving the health of children in the metropolitan St. Louis area. A particular word of thanks to the Rev. Jerry W. Paul, president of the Deaconess Foundation, and to Dr. Nesa

Joseph, vice president for administration, both of whom have dedicated countless hours to health ministry through parish nursing, health administration, health philanthropy, and other faith-based efforts to eliminate health disparities and improve community health. Thanks also to the wonderful staff of Deaconess Parish Nurse Ministries, LLC, which includes the International Parish Nurse Resource Center: Mary Ann Brischetto, Maureen Daniels, Karen Howe, Gayle Mason, Eileen McGartland, Susan Miller, Marilyn Price, Sharon Salerno, Mary Slutz,, and Dr. Andrea West, as well as each and every one of the Deaconess parish nurses serving the metropolitan St. Louis area. Thanks also to Eden Theological Seminary, our home in the world, and to all of our partner congregations and faith-based organizations.

Finally, thanks be to God for the vision and faithfulness of clergy, parish nurses, and others who seek tirelessly to bring healing and wholeness to all.

 *part one*

CALLED TO HEALTH MINISTRY

SERMON

one · MOVED BY AUTO RICKSHAW

> *On the way to Jerusalem Jesus was going through the region between Samaria and Galilee. As he entered a village, ten lepers approached him. Keeping their distance, they called out, saying, "Jesus, Master, have mercy on us!" When he saw them, he said to them, "Go and show yourselves to the priests." And as they went, they were made clean. Then one of them, when he saw that he was healed, turned back, praising God with a loud voice. He prostrated himself at Jesus' feet and thanked him. And he was a Samaritan. Then Jesus asked, "Were not ten made clean? But the other nine, where are they? Was none of them found to return and give praise to God except this foreigner?" Then he said to him, "Get up and go on your way; your faith has made you well."*
>
> **Luke 17:11–19**

A few years ago, my husband, two kids, and I traveled to India. We went to Bangalore, a city in the middle of the country, where Steve taught at United Theological Seminary for three months. The kids and I did schoolwork together each morning, and afternoons I spent working on a book and visiting local churches and hospitals.

Each morning around 11:00, after a couple of hours of homework, the kids and I went for an outing. Sometimes this involved walking to the library courtyard for a small cup of steaming hot tea—called "chai." This tea was served from bicycle by a man known as the "chaiwalla."

Sometimes our outing involved a walk. Now, this was no small feat since crossing the street in a city of 6.5 million filled with motorcycles, cars, and cows can be challenging. Especially when everyone drives on the left! Other times our outings involved going across town for shopping or sightseeing, in an auto rickshaw.

Let me tell you a little bit about an auto rickshaw. You've probably seen rickshaws with men pulling a little passenger cart behind them. Auto rickshaws are similar, but have a small motor, like a golf cart. An auto rickshaw can hold a couple of adults and a couple of kids. The number of passengers can go up from there, depending upon how cozy one is willing to get.

Auto rickshaws have several advantages: they are a little faster than walking, and they're cheap. Plus, the drivers generally know where they are going, and if you pay them to wait, they will bring you home. We became friends with a couple of drivers—two Muslim brothers named Haleen and Mohammed. We would arrange in advance to meet one or the other, and they would take us where we wanted to go, wait for us, load up our packages, and get us safely back. Mohammed even came to the airport with us, where our children hugged him goodbye and blessed him with the name "Uncle."

But riding in an auto rickshaw also has several disadvantages. First of all, auto rickshaws are closed on top and behind. During the monsoon season—most of the time we were there—the rain comes in through the open sides. They get very wet, and so do the passengers.

Second, because they are open, the smells and the grime of the city are right up close and personal. You can taste the pollution and the dust of dirt and dung blowing through the air.

And finally—did I mention these things are open??—the *passengers* are open to the city, too. When the auto rickshaw stops for a light, beggars come up from behind and reach in front of the passengers. John and Sophie and I would be sitting there and, suddenly, the bandaged hand of a leper would be thrust into our faces.

Hard to imagine, in this day and age, the same disease that Jesus encountered in his lifetime, two thousand years ago. But the lepers are still there. Crouched outside the church, by the side of the road, as people arrive for services. Standing along the roadside, calling for help, calling for hope.

In 1951, a young Indian man named Sadan traveled from his home by bus to the city of Vellore. He had heard that there was a doctor there named Paul Brand, who was able to treat people living with leprosy. On the bus, Sadan was subject to the usual: cruel stares, insults, gestures of disgust and revulsion. But he was glad to have been allowed to stay on the bus, for often lepers were thrown off in fear. Dorothy Clarke Wilson, who tells his story, writes, "When he arrived in Vellore, he was directed to the Medical College, about four miles away. He tried to take [another] bus, but the driver noticed his hands and bandaged feet and ordered him to get off. It was a hot day. Sadan was tired, his clothes rumpled, the dust of the journey ground into his pores. By the time he reached the college grounds the discharge from his ulcerated feet, seeping through the bandages, was leaving wet marks where he walked.

Outside the entrance to the college office building he met a sweet-faced woman, who, someone had told him, was Mrs. Paul Brand.

"'Pardon me.' He was careful from long experience not to step too close. 'I am looking for Dr. Brand.'

"The woman did not draw away, though Sadan was sure she had noticed his hands and feet. She explained that Dr. Brand was away on a trip, but he would be back in a day or two, and if Sadan wanted to find some place to stay in Vellore and return tomorrow . . ."

"He tried not to show his overwhelming disappointment. Then, as he turned hopelessly away, she called him back, 'You—you can find a place to stay, can't you?'

"Turning again, he found that [Margaret Brand] had moved toward him, her blue eyes looking straight into his face. And suddenly Sadan wanted to cry. For years no woman had looked at him like that, not with fear or revulsion or even pity, but with concern, as if she cared about him as another human being. And before he knew it he was telling her about the trip, the bus incident, and how impossible it would be for him to find lodging in the town. He could scarcely believe what followed. She took him home with her. She made him a comfortable bed on the verandah. She brought him food and sat and talked with him. He stayed there for three days, feeling wanted, respected, yes, even loved like a human being."

"It was late at night when [Paul] Brand returned. He had been sick. But he came to Sadan immediately, greeted him kindly, examined his hands and feet. There was a good chance, he told [Sadan], that even after all these years the ulcers might be healed because, as he believed, it was not leprosy that caused them, but walking and improper use. And the claw hands, bad though they were, could be made useful again by operations which he had tried and found successful. Sadan would be able once more to bend and straighten his fingers, to hold tools, to write, to convey food to his mouth with normal gesture. . . . They would start on his rehabilitation [in the morning]. . . . And for the first time in years Sadan [slept] well, not only because in his hopelessness he had found hope but even more because in his friendlessness he had found friends. He had been treated like a man again."[1]

It is the church in India that has cared for the lepers. Dr. Paul Brand, a doctor at Christian Medical College in Vellore, was a surgeon who operated on hands deformed by leprosy. That hospital has grown to one of the largest medical centers in India.

It is the church in India that has cared for the sick. Almost all of the nurses and doctors in India, like Drs. Margaret and Paul Brand, have been Christians. Almost all the hospitals are Christian hospitals.

And when you come right down to it, it is the church that has started almost all the hospitals in the world, most of the nursing schools, and most of the medical schools. The church heard the words of Jesus—"I was hungry and you gave me food, I was thirsty and you gave me something to drink, I was a stranger and you welcomed me, I was naked and you gave me clothing, I was sick and you took care of me, I was in prison and you visited me. . . . Truly I tell you, just as you did it to one of the least of these who are members of my family, you did it to me." (Matt. 25:35–36, 40).

The church continues its healing work today. You remember the accidents, the illnesses, the sufferings that have occurred here, in this community, among your own. You visited, you comforted, you fed, you blessed. You prayed, and you brought healing hope.

Sadan was helped by the Brands. His surgeries and treatment were successful. He married a fellow patient, became a clerk in a tuberculosis sanatorium, and together with his wife raised a healthy son. And he returned to give thanks. When Dorothy Clarke Wilson decided to write the remarkable story of the Brands and their work at Vellore, she turned to Sadan, who responded with eagerness and gratitude.

It doesn't happen very often that a person with leprosy would reach out and find a savior. I'm afraid we, from the rickshaw, were not able to restore the deformed hands we saw. But sometimes, it happens. Two thousand years ago, Jesus was there for the lepers at the side of a road to Jerusalem. Sometimes people are moved to start a hospital, to go to nursing school, to visit the sick. And sometimes people return from their healing to give God thanks.

The church continues its work of praise and thanksgiving today. We give thanks for the Spirit of God that will never let go. We praise the living, loving God. We celebrate God's goodness, despite the rain, despite the pain. We know that there is always—always—always a tomorrow and that God is the one who awaits us there.

And, *always*, the Spirit of God goes with us. We are never alone. Samaritan or Galilean. Jew or Gentile. In sickness and in health. We are embodied spirits, surrounded by the love of God that will not let us go. Thanks be to God, now, and forevermore. Amen.

SERMON

two · **NO JOY FOR YOU?!**

The spirit of the Sovereign God is upon me, because God has anointed me; God has sent me to bring good news to the oppressed, to bind up the brokenhearted, to proclaim liberty to the captives, and release to the prisoners; to proclaim the year of the Lord's favor, and the day of vengeance of our God; to comfort all who mourn; to provide for those who mourn in Zion—to give them a garland instead of ashes, the oil of gladness instead of mourning, the mantle of praise instead of a faint spirit. They will be called oaks of righteousness, the planting of the Lord, to display his glory.

Isaiah 61:1–3

Good tidings I bring to you, of great joy.

Well, joy for Jay. Jay Grinney, that is, the CEO of HealthSouth, a for-profit hospital chain. Jay earned $2.6 million dollars during 2006 in total compensation, according to the Securities and Exchange Commission. That's $1266 per hour.

Even more joyful was Michael B. McCallister, the CEO of Humana, Inc., a health-care insurance company. He received $5.8 million in compensation that year. That's almost $2,800 per hour.

But Michael is not as joyful as Trevor Fetter, CEO of Tenet Healthcare Corporation, who received $9.5 million. That's more than $4,500 per hour, nearly double what Michael McAllister made.

Even better news for Jay, Michael, and Trevor are that these figures were reported under a more modest method the SEC now uses for calculating executive pay. If they were still reporting the way they did in 2005, these CEOs' combined take would have been calculated closer to $22 million.

Now, let me tell you about Helen and Bob. They are members of a small church in a small rural community in southern Indiana. Bob worked at a small factory near their home, and he had planned to retire at age sixty-five. At about age sixty, Bob was diagnosed with lung cancer, despite never having smoked. That was a chilling diagnosis, but Helen and Bob both had the comfort of knowing that they had good health insurance through his union job.

What Bob and Helen didn't know was that Bob's treatment would quickly run up costs beyond the limits of the policy. Soon Helen faced not only the prospect of Bob's dying, but also the probable loss of her home to bankruptcy.

It was only because Bob's physician was married to one of the most tenacious parish nurses known to humankind that the hospital billing department agreed to write off the overrun to "charity care." Helen lost her husband, but she is still living in her home. Good news of great joy? Well, maybe.

Dr. Jim Kimmey, president and CEO of the Missouri Foundation for Health, one of the countries largest health foundations, calls underinsurance health care's dirty little secret. Well, it certainly is *one* of them.

America is the only developed country in the world that does not provide quality medical care to all its citizens. It is the only developed country without an emphasis on preventative care. The only developed country in the world that does not recognize the UN Declaration of Human Rights, which states in article 25.1 that "Everyone has the right to a standard of living adequate for the health and well-being of himself and of his family, including food, clothing, housing and medical care and necessary social services, and the right to security in the event of unemployment, sickness, disability, widowhood, old age or other lack of livelihood in circumstances beyond his control."

Friends, let's look back at our scripture text. It comes from the time when the Judeans were returning home from captivity in Babylon, about 2,500 years ago. Attributed to a follower of the Second Isaiah, this text from the Third Isaiah addresses people who had undergone tremendous struggle. The writer affirms, "The spirit of the Sovereign God is upon me, because God has anointed me; God has sent me to bring good news to the oppressed." It is also the text used in Luke 4 to show us that Jesus, too, was a prophet who cared about the restoration of his people.

Babylonian captivity. I believe we are there again, both literally and figuratively. We are literally in Babylon as American troops serve in a war in Iraq, the new name for that land. And, working with parish nurses, daily I hear stories that attest that we are figuratively being held captive by a health system that excludes millions, bankrupts millions, and keeps millions in jobs they despise but need for health insurance. Doctors are held captive by reimbursement plans that penalize them for spending more than seven or eight minutes with patients. Nurses are held captive by staffing patterns that keep them working longer shifts, with more and sicker patients for whom to care. Churches are being held captive by health insurance costs that prevent them from being able to call full-time pastors.

Yes, the writer of this scripture was *anointed* to bring good tidings to the afflicted,

> *sent* to bind up the brokenhearted,
> *urged* to proclaim liberty to the captives,
> *mandated* to open the prison for those who were bound.

As was Jesus.
As are we.
We are:

> *anointed* to comfort all who mourn,
> *sent* to bring the oil of gladness,
> *urged* to give a garland instead of ashes.
> *mandated* to wear a mantle of praise instead of a faint spirit.

So, let me tell you some good news. It is about a Christian who felt called to bring healing to his community. Tommy Douglas was born in Scotland in 1904 and moved to Canada six years later. As a boy, he suffered a leg injury that required surgery. His family was unable to afford the cost of the operation, so he faced probable amputation of his leg. A physician agreed to perform the operation without charge as a chance to teach his students about the procedure.

Later, Tommy became a Baptist pastor in Weyburn, saskatchewan, where he saw members of his congregation fall prey to the same financial barriers to care. Rev. Douglas felt that it was his role as a Christian to bring access to health care to all. He became active in politics and eventually became the premier of Saskatchewan. Through his leadership, universal health care became the norm in his province in 1962 and four years later in all of Canada. This was achieved over the searing opposition of those with a stake in the health care status quo.

Tommy was recently voted the "greatest Canadian of all time." He brought good tidings to the afflicted, the oil of gladness, and a mantle of praise. The Rev. Thomas Clement Douglas, along with many other church members and community leaders, proclaimed liberty to the captives.

Friends, we too are made for liberty, not for captivity. We are made for courage, not for despair. We live in a land full of people looking to Starbucks for sustenance, not to the Savior for vision and hope.

O Come, O Come Emmanuel
And ransom captive Israel
That mourns in lonely exile here
Until the son of God appear.
Rejoice! Rejoice! Emmanuel shall come to you, O Israel.[1]

The church, my friends, bring good tidings every day, through its news services and presses. The church brings good tidings through support for new ministries and new congregations. The church brings good news through ministries of healing and wholeness, around the country and around the world. And together, my friends, we can do all things through Christ who strengthens us. So let us look again to the coming of Christ for this new day, for our own time, for the challenges of our day.

REFLECTION

three · **KIDNEY STONES AND OTHER LEARNING EXPERIENCES**

For the hurt of my poor people I am hurt, I mourn, and dismay has taken hold of me. Is there no balm in Gilead? Is there no physician there? Why then has the health of my poor people not been restored?

Jeremiah 8:21–22

The poor souls who live or work with me on a daily basis know that recently I had extracorporeal shock wave lithotripsy to remove a kidney stone. If you read the sermon just before this reflection, you will know how lucky I was to have had the health insurance to pay for this procedure.

Now, the term "extracorporeal" suggests that the intervention occurs outside one's body, and it actually does. But the process certainly left me wondering about "noninvasive procedures." I was a little taken aback (OK, a *lot* taken aback!!) by the intensity and duration of the discomfort. Like most people my age, I have had my share of minor surgeries and medical interventions. But this experience opened the world of pain for me in a whole new way.

Dr. Paul Brand was a physician who pioneered reconstructive surgery for people with leprosy in Vellore, India. Working in the 1940s and '50s, he discovered that most people lost fingers or toes due to secondary infections, not because leprosy ravaged their extremities. Damage to the nerves from the virus left them unable to feel pain from small injuries. Without care for the original, minor traumas, they were susceptible to further, debilitating damage.

Dr. Brand, in a lecture to the British Medical Association in Oxford, said, "It is clear how important pain must be in the whole pattern of the survival of living organisms composed of many cells. As soon as pain is lost there seems to be a loss also of that body consciousness which makes every part share the success or failure of the whole. It is clear that once pain is lost, different parts of the body may revert to competition with each other. Thus, our very survival depends on pain."[1]

In the church, as the body of Christ, we must open our eyes and our hearts to the pain of our brothers and sisters. "Survival of the fittest" should not be a motto for people of faith. Indeed, the Apostle Paul wrote to the church in Corinth, "Those parts of the body that seem to be weaker are indispensable" (1 Cor. 12:22 NIV).

Parish nurses and health ministers are uniquely positioned to see the pain of the hungry, the lonely, the sorrowing, and the sick. They are uniquely placed, not only to bring help on a case-by-case basis, but to assist with change. Rev. Eileen Lindner of the National Council of Churches, recently reminded their Health Task Force that faith communities played an instrumental role in the creation of the food stamp program, moving aid for the hungry beyond soup kitchens. We have other opportunities to effect change today.

So thank God both for pain and for comfort. The movement of the Spirit is opening eyes to suffering, and it is calling forth remarkable responses of compassion and justice.

REFLECTION

four · MYSTICS, VISIONARIES, AND HEALERS

*Before I formed you in the womb I knew you,
and before you were born I consecrated you.*

Jeremiah 1:5a

When I was reading Barbara Dossey's book, *Florence Nightingale: Mystic, Visionary, Healer,* something nagged at me, but I couldn't put my finger on it. Then it dawned on me: she was very much like a parish nurse! Here was Florence, who knew from childhood that she had a call from God to care for others, and who absorbed as much knowledge as she could about the workings of the human body. Here was a young woman who went to the church in Kaiserswerth, Germany, to take Deaconess training to become a nurse. Here was a determined woman who, given limited resources, turned those resources into hope for ill and poor governesses in Britain, and later for an entire army during the Crimean War.

I see parish nurses all around with limited resources but incredible vision and energy. I see women of faith, from many different theological backgrounds, who are working in poor neighborhoods, seeking to care for those who have limited access to health-care services. I see women who, like Florence, can move between economic classes with ease, and who can change the lives of all.

Parish nurses must have a strong sense of vocation—there is no one to tell them exactly what to do. They need to determine what needs to be done and do it, or arrange for it to be done. Parish nurses need to be brave, for there is no end to the suffering and pain they see. Parish nurses need to be creative in proactively addressing the needs of each community in which they find themselves, and they need to be vigilant in staying on the cutting edge of their profession.

There is a wonderful missionary hymn written by Howard A. Walter, who died at the age of thirty-five while working for the YMCA in India. The first verse follows:

I would be true,
for there are those who trust me,
I would be pure,
for there are those who care;
I would be strong,
for there is much to suffer,
I would be brave,
for there is much to dare.[1]

We live in a world where faith-filled, visionary healers are needed as much as ever. Parish nurses are following in those footsteps well!

REFLECTION

five · MINISTRY LOVES COMPANY

*And God has appointed in the church first apostles,
second prophets, third teachers; then deeds of power, then gifts
of healing, forms of assistance, forms of leadership,
various kinds of tongues.*

1 Corinthians 12:28

In his book *Ministry Loves Company*, John Galloway Jr. shares ideas for surviving ministry. He writes, "[W]e have become a bunch of chickens. We hassle and whine and manipulate, often making a big deal of minor issues. We do not seem to have the courage to lead on the issues that matter most. As a group, we in the clergy do not have a compelling sense of vision. We have lost the capacity to dream about what is possible."[1]

Edwina Gateley has not lost this capacity. A person of faith, she sees her work as ministry and focuses on what is important. Her ministry has included traveling to Uganda in 1964, where she started a school for girls. It has since grown into one of the largest in the area. In 1969, Edwina began the "Volunteer Missionary Movement," which has sent 1,700 missionaries from the United Kingdom and the United States to work in crosscultural missions of developing countries. In 1983, she had the courage to open a house of hospitality and nurture in Chicago for women in prostitution. Later in life, she felt called to adopt a child.

Ministry loves company. We are given vision for ministry to which we are invited to respond. Shall we respond with courage?

What is your vision for ministry in these days? How do you respond to God's call upon your life? Ministry loves company.

REFLECTION

six · THE HIDDEN COUNTRY WITHIN

> *For surely I know the plans I have for you, says God, plans for your welfare and not for harm, to give you a future with hope. Then when you call upon me and come and pray to me, I will hear you. When you search for me, you will find me; if you seek me with all your heart, I will let you find me, says God, and I will restore your fortunes and gather you from all the nations and all the places where I have driven you, says God, and I will bring you back to the place from which I sent you into exile.*
>
> **Jeremiah 29:11–14**

Recently, I had the opportunity to spend an hour over coffee with a young mother of a special needs teenager, talking about her family's health-care situation. Their son had a degenerative neurological condition, and she had needed to quit her job to stay home and take care of him. Money was very tight, but at least they had her husband's health insurance coverage. This was a comfort, until he lost his job. Then they tried to make a go of it through freelance work in their respective professions, but there was no way they could afford any health insurance coverage without being part of an employee group, particularly with a child as severely disabled as theirs. Their son qualified for the state children's health insurance program, but once they had him enrolled, they had difficulty finding physicians with the expertise they needed who would accept this form of "socialized" medicine. She told me she was begging, begging, always begging for the care he needed. The bills were a constant worry.

At the International Parish Nurse Resource Center, we are in the process of updating our curriculum for parish nurse basic preparation. Our Educational Partner in Canada, Inter-Church Health Ministries, is working on a Canadian version of this curriculum, because some items simply are not applicable there. For example, in the module on the role of the parish nurse as advocate, telling people that there are 47 million uninsured citizens in the country would be inaccurate. There are no uninsured citizens in Canada.

In fact, if all Canadians lost their health insurance today, that entire population of 33.4 million would still be fewer people than the number of uninsured Americans in 2009. It is as if we have a hidden country of uninsured citizens right here among us.

Paul, speaking to the church at Ephesus, reminded them, "You are . . . fellow citizens with God's people and members of God's household" (Eph. 2:19 NIV). As people of God, can we let our fellow citizens suffer, even die, for lack of access to care?

We remember the words of God to the prophet Jeremiah, speaking to God's people living in exile in Babylon, hidden in another country: "'For I know the plans I have for you,' declares the LORD, 'plans to prosper you and not to harm you, plans to give you a hope and a future'" (Jer. 29:11 NIV).

Let's claim that future and that hope, for all God's people!

CALLED TO HEALTH MINISTRY
Discussion Questions

1. Jesus called us to preach, teach, *and* heal. What is our congregation already doing related to the healing ministries of the church?
2. Most hospitals around the world were started by the church. How do those health systems relate to the healing mission of the church today?
3. There seems to be a hierarchy of financial reimbursement for care, with more money available for care of physical illnesses than for mental health care. Why do you think that mental health care does not receive parity under the majority of health insurance plans?
4. Do you see health-related needs in the church today that could be addressed through growing the health ministry of the congregation?
5. Are there areas of caring outreach in which the church can offer unique gifts?

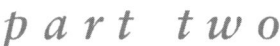 *part two*

ACCESS TO HEALTH CARE

SERMON

seven · IF RELIGION WAS A THING THAT MONEY COULD BUY

> *"If religion was a thing that money could buy,
> the rich would live, and the poor would die..."*
>
> **American folk song**

During the first year of study at Eden Seminary, students are required to work in a mission setting, such as a jail, homeless shelter, after-school program, or hospital. Professor Marilyn Stavenger was the director of Field Education when I studied there, and she assigned me to St. Louis Regional Hospital, which was a consolidation of the former St. Louis City and County Hospitals—the public hospital, that is, for poor people and people without health insurance.

I didn't want to go there. I wanted to go to the jail or someplace else safe. I wanted to be safe from the grave danger of seeing needles and blood. You see, my mother was a nurse, and I had seen her textbooks. I wasn't interested. I was going to be a minister, and this hospital thing would be only a hoop to jump through on the way to the pulpit, thank you very much.

But let me tell you a little of what I saw there. I saw a young woman, probably in her early twenties, who had kidney stones. She had simply needed to have the kidney stones pulverized through extracorporeal shock wave lithotripsy, a short, noninvasive procedure that has the normal, healthy patient going home in a couple of hours. In any other hospital, they would have had the equipment to do this. However, at Regional, the only treatment option was surgery the old fashioned way—the whole nine yards of cutting into the kidney and taking out the stone. There were complications. She had been in the hospital for nearly a month by the time I saw her. Did I mention that she was a college student? Studying nursing? She certainly seemed to know a great deal about what her treatment options had been and about her current condition. Did I mention that she was a single mom? Her toddler son had been staying with friends for that entire time, wondering why his mommy was still in the hospital. Did I mention that she didn't have health insurance? A student nurse with no health insurance. There she was: a young woman, a single mom, a student nurse, who probably chose between food and child care for her child or health insurance, as she was working her way through nursing school.

Let me tell you about another patient I saw. I saw a young man, probably in his thirties, who appeared nearly shrouded in the white hospital sheets. His emaciated body was covered with nearly translucent, blue skin. He wasn't getting much oxygen, despite a number of attempts to change that. He was in isolation, with a grief-stricken family huddled around him, and a frightened friend hovering outside the door. This young man was one of the first AIDS patients I saw, and I will never forget the terror in the eyes of that young man who was dying before us all, in the prime of his life. Did I mention that he had been employed until his hospitalization? Did I mention that he didn't have any health insurance?

Finally, let me tell you about one other man. This somewhat older man was probably in his mid-to-late fifties. He was lying down in a bed that had been pushed near a window, all alone in a room. I walked in and we exchanged a few words. As we talked, my inexperienced seminary student eyes noticed that the shape under the sheets was a little different than most of the other bed-ridden shapes. This man was a patient who had been living for some time with diabetes. He had lost both legs, and both arms, to the ravages of the disease. I was talking to a man whose body had been reduced to a head and a torso. Did I mention that he had been working until his first amputation? Did I mention that he was now living in poverty? Did I mention that he had no health insurance?

If religion was a thing that money could buy,
the rich would live and the poor would die . . .

- At the time of the 2000 U.S. Census, the number of the uninsured in this country was 41.2 million people.[1]

- In 2008, a conservative estimate of the number of the uninsured was more than 47 million.[2]

- Nearly one-quarter of the uninsured were children,[3] and 55 percent of the uninsured were under the age of thirty-five.[4] That's the nursing student, and the young man with AIDS.

- More than 90 percent of the uninsured had some attachment to the workforce.[93]

SERMON: If Religion Was a Thing That Money Could Buy

⁵ That's the young man with AIDS and the older man, who had been working when he was first diagnosed with diabetes. Neither of them is able to work any longer.

- The National Coalition on Health Care recently reported that, in 2007, this country spent 17 percent of its gross domestic product on health-care expenditures. Seventeen percent of our GDP means $2.4 trillion dollars spent on health care in just one year. That amounts to $7,900 per person.⁶

Now, what would your congregation do if you had $7,900 per person to spend? At my home congregation, a medium-sized congregation, we would have an annual budget of about $2.3 million. We could have a staff of two dozen or more. We could hire several full-time pastors, several church musicians, administrators, and pastoral counselors, and we could fund a clinic with a physician, a nurse practitioner, a midwife, and a parish nurse. All paid, all full-time. That's a lot of money.

So, why are we in this situation? Let's blame it on the nuns in Wisconsin! The sisters at St. Joseph Hospital in Chippewa Falls, Wisconsin, to be exact. In 1897, these women religious thought it would be a good idea if the loggers they saw at their hospital all shared the cost of illness care. Then individuals would not be burdened with large medical bills. For $7.50 a year, the loggers could buy a voucher that would cover care at fourteen cooperating hospitals. This was when a week in the hospital cost about five dollars, and you'd often get back change.

But probably those sisters aren't entirely responsible for this state of affairs. Maybe we should blame it on employers.

During and following WWII, factories needed to attract and keep workers, and so they started offering health insurance as a benefit. In the 1960s the government jumped in to cover the two largest groups who didn't have employers—the retired and the nonworking poor. Medicare was formed to provide health insurance for medical care of the elderly, and Medicaid was started as a health-care safety net for the poor. All this increased revenue increased demand for services, and it meant more funds for development of technology and drugs.

When our hospitals were being founded there was precious little medical technology, and very few drugs. There were no antibiotics—none. Technology, such as the use of X-rays, was in its infancy. And speaking of infants, there were no neonatal units, not even a single baby incubator. It wasn't until a hundred years ago—1904—that the first baby incubators were displayed to the world at Deaconess Hospital, as part of the St. Louis World's Fair.

Ok, it's probably not really the employers' fault; they were just trying to help their workers. So, let's blame the doctors.

Doctors used to make house calls, and those were much cheaper. Hospitals were started for the destitute. Those who could afford to pay for a doctor stayed at home and the doctor came to them. The doctor would bring his little black bag with medicine like "Elixir Pan-Peptic," or "Lithiated Sorghum Compound S & D." Many of the early medications contained a fair amount of alcohol—understandably since there were as yet no antibiotics for treatment of infectious diseases, no modern anesthesia to remove pain during surgery.

One hundred years ago a doctor was paid the same a clergyperson. Before the Flexner Report was released in 1910, which radically standardized medical education,[7] many physicians had far less formal education than clergy. Some gave haircuts on the side to supplement their income.

Medical students now often pay more than $100,000 to get through medical school. To remain in their practice, they pay many thousands of dollars in malpractice insurance on an annual basis, and some are leaving the field because of soaring premiums. Their chosen profession can put them in harm's way, cavorting with disease and death. Doctors often are forced to neglect their families to provide care to their patients, and are caught in the middle of the health-care system.

They are caught in the middle, because the patients aren't really their customers. The health insurance companies are—they provide the patients. So, all this health-care mess is the insurance companies' fault, right?

Well, not all the insurance companies are cut from the same cloth. For example, many denominations have health plans for their ordained clergy and other ministry professionals. The United

Church of Christ's health insurance plan costs around $12,000 for a family at the present time. And it is hard to get on it if you have pre-existing conditions, unless you are a brand-new pastor. The UCC health plan is working very hard to provide health insurance coverage because of the rising costs of hospitalizations. And for another reason: insurance boards like the UCC health plan, among others, are paying a huge amount of money for prescription drug coverage.

So, maybe we should blame it on Rev. August Hermann Francke, a seventeenth-century Pietist in Halle, Germany, who funded part of his extensive outreach ministry of education and social services through the proceeds of a pharmacy he started. The profits from the sale of drugs were enough to fund a lot of outreach, and drug companies today are following his footsteps, although probably not as Francke would have liked. The *New York Times* recently reported that the cost for the AIDS drug Norvir had increased significantly. Last year, Norvir cost about $1,500 for an annual supply. This past January, Abbott Laboratories raised the cost to $7,800 per year, an increase of over $6,000. Abbott Laboratories said they were doing this because they needed the money for research and couldn't get it from other countries. They couldn't get it from other countries because the cost of drugs is regulated elsewhere.

So, blame the profits of the pharmaceutical business on the good Herr Pastor Francke. But he used his money for seminaries and schools and hospitals. The Deaconess Sisters and other good church folks, our ancestors, started other hospitals. Maybe we should blame this mess on the hospitals.

When the Deaconess Sisters started running Deaconess Hospital in St. Louis, Sister Katherine Haack, Sister Superior, was paid $.50 per day, or $182.50 a year. When Rev. Jens was hired as the first Superintendent nine years later, his salary was more than three times higher, at $600 a year, and was raised 25 percent the very next year. Now, some hospital executives are *still* making a lot of money. The average midpoint salary for a CEO of a hospital in 1997 was $303,000, and the average bonus was $61,000. The chief administrative officer of Westchester Medical Center in New York was recently criticized for taking a raise of over $200,000, making his salary nearly half a million dollars, while 292 other employees were laid off within the last year.[8] (Of course, a typical hospital president's salary is slightly lower than a typical HMO president's salary, so you don't hear HMOs complain about this.)[9]

Health insurance often reimburses providers amounts that are painfully close to the actual costs of procedures, however. This is why hospitals are closing their emergency departments. This is why they are laying off nurses and asking those who stay on to work twelve-hour shifts. This is why some health systems are building specialty hospitals. They are following bank robber Willy Sutton's rule to go where the money is. Sioux Valley Hospital in South Dakota, which is lobbying *against* specialty hospitals, estimates that it makes nearly $1,500 for a typical coronary bypass under Medicare, while it loses almost $1,800 treating a case of simple pneumonia and $2,500 on a patient with kidney failure. Who do you think is excited when elderly folks show up with pneumonia or kidney failure? Which of us is not going to be elderly some day? Only those of us who will already be dead.

What a mess! The uninsured, the underinsured, the high cost of insurance, the high cost of hospitalizations, the high cost of drugs! What *can* the church do about this?

Well, Jesus called us to preach, teach, and heal. That is why we have a sermon here in this pulpit every single week. Even when the pastor is gone, she makes arrangements for somebody else to preach. It is a gospel mandate.

This is why we teach—we have adult education and Sunday school every week. We don't leave Christian education and preaching the gospel solely to others—we feel there is a significant role for the church to play in this regard. But the church also has a significant role to play in fulfilling the gospel mandate to heal. Lately, the church's role in healing has shrunk to serving as guinea pigs in ambiguous prayer studies and as ambivalent observers of faith healings.

This is no longer 1850. Medical education and nursing education are much more technically sophisticated than when the church was starting hospitals. Hospitals are no longer staffed by church volunteers who bring in soup for the sick. However, the church has a moral obligation—a gospel call—to participate in healing.

The church needs to shout out the good news about wellness

and prevention! Only 3 percent of the trillions of dollars spent on health care are spent on prevention. We can advocate for wellness—every week we walk in here and sit. Well, what if churches were places where walking happened?

We can advocate for all working people, and the poor, to receive the health care they need. There is no excuse for us to spend nearly $8,000 per person, yet leave some out. The un- and underinsured will still get care anyway, only it will be ahead of us in line at the emergency room. They will receive charity care for treatment of diseases that might have been more successfully and cost-effectively treated earlier, if they had had insurance to cover routine testing and regular office visits.

We can write letters or make phone calls to our elected officials, telling them that we want our state to be a state where health plans are available to all. We can vote. We shouldn't be arguing over whether health care is a right or a privilege. According to Jesus, caring for the sick is neither: it's a commandment.

There are all kinds of church-related health programs, like health clinics and parish nursing, lay health workers and Stephen's Ministries, through which the church can make a difference. And this is only the tip of the iceberg of how we can be involved in healing and wholeness. The Jewish faith community is speaking these days of *Shleimut*—wholeness—and they have begun opening healing centers around the country. The Islamic Faith Community says "God is greater" and is busy training physicians and nurses who are sensitive to their own traditions.

We started this mess. We really did. We meant well, as the church, as clergy, as deaconesses, as doctors, as nurses, as lay people. We wanted people to be well, so we worked to create this system. Here we are. But we cannot throw up our hands and say, now, someone else fix it! Who else will do it? We are the people of this country. We are the people to whom Jesus says today, "Feed my sheep and heal the sick!"

So let us not turn our backs on Jesus's mandate to preach, teach, *and* heal. Let us not turn from our marvelous heritage as people of faith to be leaders in healing.

SERMON

eight · REWRITING YOUR FUTURE

Jesus said to the disciples, "There was a rich man who had a manager, and charges were brought to him that this man was squandering his property. So he summoned him and said to him, 'What is this that I hear about you? Give me an account of your management, because you cannot be my manager any longer.' Then the manager said to himself, 'What will I do, now that my master is taking the position away from me? I am not strong enough to dig, and I am ashamed to beg. I have decided what to do so that, when I am dismissed as manager, people may welcome me into their homes.' So, summoning his master's debtors one by one, he asked the first, 'How much do you owe my master?' He answered, 'A hundred jugs of olive oil.' He said to him, 'Take your bill, sit down quickly, and make it fifty.' Then he asked another, 'And how much do you owe?' He replied, 'A hundred containers of wheat.' He said to him, 'Take your bill and make it eighty.' And his master commended the dishonest manager because he had acted shrewdly; for the children of this age are more shrewd in dealing with their own generation than are the children of light. And I tell you, make friends for yourselves by means of dishonest wealth so that when it is gone, they may welcome you into the eternal homes."

Luke 16:1-9

The Chilean writer Isabel Allende has written such novels as *The House of the Spirits* and *The Stories of Eva Luna*, mining her past for stories. Allende also has written several memoirs. One of the most poignant is entitled *Paula*, written for and about her daughter, who was in a coma from complications from a rare neurological disorder. Paula died in 1992, three years before the book's publication.

A more recent memoir is *My Invented Country: A Nostalgic Journey through Chile*, in which Allende describes her native land for fellow citizens in her new home—the United States. Most U.S. citizens have never been to South America and many would be hard-pressed to locate Chile on a world map.

Chile, Allende tells us, extends from the middle of the west coast of South America to the southern reaches of the continent and beyond in a slice to the South Pole. She says that Chile is *in* South America, but close to Europe. It took the side of Britain during Britain's war with Argentina over the Falkland Islands. Some of the best German food in the world can be found in the southern provinces.

Allende readily acknowledges, however, that her description of Chile comes from what she has retained in her memory. She has not lived there for more than thirty years, after a coup brought Pinochet to power in 1973. As first cousin, once removed, of ousted President Salvador Allende, she found herself targeted for assassination.

Fleeing to Argentina and later to America, her writing takes her back, back, back. She uncovers and re-invents stories from her past and from her memories. When she did live in Chile, it was mostly as a child and young adult. She rewrote her past as memory brought it back in *My Invented Country*.

In telling about the food of her country, for example, she includes this wonderful description of a regular family gathering:

> A typical luncheon at my grandfather's house began with stick-to-the-ribs fried *empanadas*, meat pies with onion, which can provoke heartburn in the healthiest eater; then came a *cazuela*, a raise-the-dead soup of meat, corn, potatoes, and vegetables, followed by a succulent seafood *chupe* that flooded the house with its delicious aroma, and to end, we had a selection of irresistible desserts, which always included a tarte of *manjar blanco* or *dulce de leche*, a milk-based caramel (my aunt Cupertino's legendary recipe)—all accompanied by our fatal *pisco* sours and several bottles of good red wine that had been aged for years in the family cellar. Before we left, we were given a tablespoon of milk of magnesia. This dosage was increased by five when an adult birthday was being celebrated: we children didn't merit such

deference. I never heard the word cholesterol mentioned. My parents, who are over eighty, consume ninety eggs, a quart of cream, a pound of butter, and four pounds of cheese per week. They are healthy and lively as little kids.[1]

Eighty-year-olds—who eat ninety eggs a week? A quart of cream, a pound of butter, and four pounds of cheese per week? Healthy and lively as little kids? Could this be true? In the word of one of our kids' favorite children's books, "I don't think so, Sammy!" But Allende has invented—rewritten—her country in a way that engages and gratifies the reader, and she makes her case that it was a wonderful place to live as she unearths stories to share.

Like the manager in the biblical text we read today, Allende's rewriting of the bottom line helps both parties in the transaction. The writer manages her ghosts, blesses her past, and expands her future. The reader is spared a dry rendition of social studies: "Chile is a country of 16.6 million people that produces a third of the world's copper and is the fifth largest exporter of wine. . . ." Allende's stories connect readers with their own invented countries in new ways through a reduction of the debt to textbook detail.

The story that Jesus told in today's scripture reading is quite straightforward. A manager has squandered his master's property and is about to be sacked. The manager calls in his master's debtors and asks them to review their bills. He directs them to rewrite future obligations to the master, cutting their debts in a way that will ingratiate them to the dishonest manager in the future. The master learns of this action and commends the manager for his shrewd behavior. Jesus ends the story by saying, "I tell you, make friends for yourselves by means of dishonest wealth, so that when it is gone, they may welcome you into the eternal homes."

But how can one make friends for oneself by means of dishonest wealth? You can't! Jesus goes on to say, "No slave can serve two masters; for a slave will either hate the one and love the other, or be devoted to the one and despise the other. You cannot serve God and wealth" (Luke 16:13).

This is an interesting parable. We believe that "you always have the poor with you." (Matt. 26:11) is literally true. And yet we believe that the saying "you cannot serve God and wealth" is metaphorical.

We believe "sell your possessions, and give the money to the poor" to be even more metaphorical!

This is also a confusing parable. Was Jesus advocating that we lie, cheat, and steal? It looks like it. This is probably one of the toughest lectionary passages in the cycle. I'm surprised they left it in, actually. Usually the hard passages are left out of the lectionary. This could be read: good job, tricking "the man." Good job, helping the "little guy." But the manager didn't reduce debts to help the little guy—he did it to help himself.

Jesus spent most of his ministry preaching, teaching, *and* healing. Healing was central of his ministry, and it seems to me that economic healing was a focus of his work. He talked about the poor and money a lot! Are economics a health issue, too?

Maybe.

In 2008, forty-seven million people had no access to health care because of economic issues.

Medical debt is the leading cause of bankruptcy in this country.

Most of those bankruptcies aren't caused by catastrophic illness or injury. These bankruptcies are generally for around $10,000 in medical bills that people put on their credit cards and cannot pay off as interest and fees keep rising.

The cost of health insurance for those who *are* covered keeps rising. The cost of covering a family on the Deaconess Foundation's health insurance plan, for example, is more than $15,000 per year. And the hourly salary of a parish nurse is only $15 per hour. We pay the cost for the employee—about $7200—and the nurse pays for her family: you do the math. Most parish nurses work only ten hours each week and do not qualify for benefits at all.

More than 40 percent of seminary students are uninsured. They fit the demographics of the largest group of the uninsured—those in the eighteen-to-thirty-five-year-old group. They are unlike the majority of uninsured, however, in that most of the uninsured in this country are working full-time.

So, take this bill, this terrible debt of medical bankruptcy, fear, and shame, and write: health care for all. All the other industrialized nations provide access to health care for all, through a single payer plan or through a panel of insurance companies. They do so at a lower cost, and often with better health-care outcomes.

Take *this* bill, the growing risk of obesity and diabetes, and write: daily PE classes for kids, bike paths for our communities, neighborhoods that are conducive to walking—peaceful, safe, pedestrian-friendly neighborhoods, throughout our cities, in every nation.

Recently, a friend of mine traveled back to visit a country he had seen before as a soldier: Vietnam. He was received with kindness and warmth everywhere he went. How is it that Americans can travel unmolested in a country where they were once the targets of military action? How can Americans travel around Germany, around Russia, around Japan? What is this thing called war and how does it fade? How is it healed? How do we bring healing?

Take this bill for war debt, and write: money for home health care, money for paid maternity leave, money for peacemaking.

You can't love God and money. But you can *use* money to make peace, to bring hope, to make friends. You can use money to work for justice, to work for an end to HIV/AIDS, TB, and malaria, to bring healing to a broken world.

As individuals, we don't really have much to gain by working for health care for all, clean water for all, peace for all. There's not much in it for us. But as Samuel Johnson said, "The true measure of a man is how he treats someone who can do him absolutely no good."

God has entrusted us with much, as managers and stewards in a world with magnificent resources. Let us use those resources to bring healing and wholeness. Let us "re-invent our country" with justice and mercy as our largest domestic products and exports. Let us manage our ghosts, and our past, and our future.

As Jesus suggests, let us copy the manager and rewrite old debts. With Jesus Christ we pray, as he taught us: forgive us our debts, as we forgive our debtors.

For God's alone is the kingdom, and the power, and the glory forever. Amen.

REFLECTION

nine · **PRAYING FOR HEALTH CARE**

> *I hope in the Lord Jesus to send Timothy to you soon, so that I may be cheered by news of you. I have no one like him who will be genuinely concerned for your welfare. All of them are seeking their own interests, not those of Jesus Christ.*
>
> **Philippians 2:19–21**

According to the Kaiser Family Foundation, 61.9 percent of working Americans now get health insurance through their employers, down from 71 percent in 1987.[1]

But maybe that's not so bad. A recent article in the *New England Journal of Medicine* stated that only 54.9 percent of U.S. adults receive recommended health care regardless of their health insurance status, gender, economic status, or ethnicity.[2]

But maybe that's not so bad, either. Lisa Sanders, M.D., once stated in *The New York Times Magazine* that at her graduation from medical school the dean said, "Half of what we teach you here is wrong—unfortunately, we don't know which half."[3]

If your chance of receiving recommended care is only slightly better than your chance of not getting it even *with* insurance, and if the recommended care might be wrong anyway, you'd better start praying.

Or maybe not. The results of a ten-year study by Dr. Herbert Benson of the Mind/Body Medical Institute and Harvard Medical School found that heart patients who knew that they were being prayed for had higher rates of complications, including heart attacks and strokes.[4]

It's enough to drive one to drink. But not soda. The average American adult drinks fifty-six gallons of soda a year, contributing to the deaths of 112,000 people annually from obesity-related causes.[5]

Perhaps we should move to Australia or to Canada where there is universal health care. A 2005 survey of adults there, however, as well as adults in Germany, New Zealand, the United Kingdom, and the United States, found that sizable shares of patients in all six countries reported safety risks, poor care coordination, and deficiencies in care for chronic conditions.[6]

We live in a world that is broken. There is no perfect way to fix all the sick and dying. We live in a world crying out for justice and healing. We live in a world with sin.

Perhaps we should be less concerned about measuring God and more concerned about assessing our complacency with lifestyles that promote illness and health systems that do not care for all. Crying out for justice for ourselves and for our neighbors is a good way to pray. It is one with a long history in most religious traditions.

We can't eliminate sin and brokenness, but we can fight against it in ourselves and in our world. As people of God, can we do less and live with ourselves at the end of the day? For sin and death do not have the last word—redemption and blessing are God's gifts to all.

REFLECTION

ten · **HEALTH CARE FOR AN ARM AND A LEG**

> *Then I heard the voice of God saying, "Whom shall I send, and who will go for us?" And I said, "Here am I; send me!"*
>
> **Isaiah 6:8**

Tim Doss drives a cement truck for an Indiana company. Or he did—for a decade, until on September 18, 2008, he was laid off. On that day, he was told, "As of midnight, your insurance is lapsed." He and his wife, Helen, already have a $3,000 bill for hospital copayments for which the creditors have come calling. The Dosses both have health conditions requiring medications, regular doctor visits, and tests. His annual checkup, required to keep his commercial driver's license, cost $300 even before he lost his insurance, and his wife, who is skipping her mammogram this year because they are uninsured, has a family history of breast cancer. Her mother died from that disease at age 56.[1]

The *Washington Post* reported that "nationwide, the number of consumers who went without prescriptions, tapped into retirement savings to pay for health care or skipped a doctor visit for themselves or a child has risen since last year, according to a survey released this summer by the Rockefeller Foundation and *Time Magazine*. One-quarter of the 2,000 respondents, for example, said they had decided not to see a doctor because of cost in 2008, up from 18 percent the year before. Ten percent said they did not take a child to the doctor for the same reason."[2]

Pat Gleich of the National Health Ministries of the Presbyterian Church (USA) wrote not very long ago:

> "For those who are bothered by the rising costs of health care and are wondering how many people are going to afford care, or if there is a feasible way to provide coverage for

the 46+ million folks who have no health insurance, you will take comfort to note that, at least for some, these rising costs have a silver, a very silver, lining. As reported on Kaisernetwork.org (January 19, 2007) 'UnitedHealth Group announced fourth-quarter earnings of $1.2 billion, in part because of the recent acquisition of PacifiCare Health Systems and business from Medicare prescription drug plans, *Reuters* reports. Revenue increased by 47% from a year earlier to about $18.16 billion, the company said.'[3]

How long, um, are we going to, um, sort of, um, talk about, um, the maybe, like, a possible, um, *problem* here?

Do you remember Tommy Douglas from an earlier chapter in this book? He was that Baptist minister who, while he was a little boy in the Canadian province of Saskatchewan, almost lost his leg to osteomyelitis because his family could not afford a surgery needed to fight the infection. A visiting surgeon operated on him for free, with the caveat that his students be allowed to observe. Later, Douglas became a Baptist clergyman and saw parishioners similarly falling through cracks in the Canadian health system of the 1940s. He decided he must do something about it, and his efforts on behalf of health care for all in his home province led to the foundation of health care coverage for the entire country.

In the United States working families have been paying greater percentages of their wages for health care. In 2008, the annual premium that a health insurer charged an employer for health coverage for a family of four was $12,700, eclipsing the gross earnings for a full-time, minimum-wage worker ($10, 712). Of course, only part of that premium is paid by the employee, but workers contributed nearly $3,400 (12 percent) more for employment-based health insurance than they did in 2007. And health insurance premiums were the fastest growing cost component for employers, threatening to eclipse profits in 2008.[4]

Even though in 2007 the United States spent 17 percent of its GDP on health care, more than other industrialized countries spent, by 2009 it still was not providing health insurance for all its citizens.[5]

Will it be the UnitedHealth companies of the world who bring health care justice to our parishioners? Will it be your pastor? Or will it be you?

REFLECTION

eleven · **DOWNSTAIRS ON A FIRST-NAME BASIS**

> *But now thus says God, who created you,*
> *O Jacob, he who formed you, O Israel:*
> *"Do not fear, for I have redeemed you;*
> *I have called you by name, you are mine."*
>
> **Isaiah 43:1**

Mark Twain once said, "Habit is habit and not to be flung out of the window by any man, but coaxed downstairs a step at a time."[1]

I am fairly good at *writing* about exercise, rest, and healthy nutrition, but I am also good at *avoiding* exercise, staying up too late, and eating too much cake. I need to be coaxed downstairs a step at a time to go for a walk. I need someone to say to me, "Step away from the cookies, and no one will get hurt." Luckily, my husband is a brave man, willing to do what needs to be done, and we have started lunchtime walks.

Rev. Dr. Granger Westberg, recalling a time when he was hospitalized, said that his wife, Helen, was his main support there, and that the chaplain helped *him* most by supporting her.[1]

Health is not a solitary endeavor. That is why the Hebrew Scriptures are filled with health laws for the community to observe together. That is why we have exercise clubs, YMCAs, and track teams. That is why we have support groups to help each other lose weight, stop smoking, and keep moving.

A conference held in Chapel Hill, North Carolina, called "The Power of Connection: Group Health Care for the 21st Century" provided further evidence for effectiveness of the group model of health promotion. Sponsored by the Centering Pregnancy and

Parenting Organization (www.centeringpregnancy.com), the conference presented data showing that using this model with prenatal care was able to reduce the level of preterm delivery by *a third*, a particularly remarkable result because it involved only two simple changes: group support and the opportunity to spend more time with health providers.[2]

Often people are greeted at the front office of a clinic with the question, "Last name?" When they get in the exam room, they are whisked through and back out the exit. Parish nurses know the people with whom they work by first name, family name, and nickname. Even more, parish nurses know what God feels about all people: "I have called you by name, you are mine."

We are not alone. We do not need to fling our habits (or ourselves) out of the window. We can coax one another down the steps, one at a time, and out the door into the beautiful sunshine of God's glorious creation (with sunscreen of at least 15 SPF).

REFLECTION

twelve · THE HARDEST WORDS

Moses said to God, "O my God, I have never been eloquent, neither in the past nor even now that you have spoken to your servant; but I am slow of speech and slow of tongue." Then God said to him, "Who gives speech to mortals? Who makes them mute or deaf, seeing or blind? Is it not I, God? Now go, and I will be with your mouth and teach you what you are to speak."

Exodus 4:10–12

Recently, the American Association of Critical Care Nurses (AACN) issued the results of a study they had cosponsored that found that in order to decrease medical errors and increase quality of care, healthcare professionals must improve interpersonal communication. According to data used in the study, 195,000 people die annually in U.S. hospitals due to medical errors. The study identified seven categories of conversations that are especially difficult, yet essential for people to master, including discussing:

1. Broken rules
2. Mistakes
3. Lack of support
4. Incompetence
5. Poor teamwork
6. Disrespect
7. Micromanagement[1]

Forty-eight percent of nurses in the study stated that they work with people who show poor clinical judgment, and 62 percent state that they have seen others taking shortcuts that could be dangerous to patients. Only 10 percent of the health-care professionals surveyed raise these issues with others, but those who do observe better patient outcomes, work harder, are more satisfied and are more committed to staying with their jobs.[2]

In parish nursing, the work that one does is seen both as a professional calling and as a ministry. Yet, even within this "double calling," one faces difficult communication issues—with other leaders in the congregation, with parishioners, with other parish nurses, and the list goes on. It is hard to raise difficult or painful issues in a place that is supposed to be "religious."

Perhaps we would do well to recall that as people of faith we have the responsibility to be both prophetic and pastoral—to speak words of truth, and to do so in love. At times we need to speak them to others, and at other times we need to hear them ourselves.

There is much brokenness in the world, but there is also much hope for new life and transformation. Remember the 10 percent who spoke up? Let's raise that number in all of our healing places.

ACCESS TO HEALTH CARE
Discussion Questions

1. Why do you think that all people in the United States do not have health insurance coverage?
2. What are some of the barriers to providing health insurance coverage to all people in this country?
3. Should doctors and other health providers be allowed to choose whether or not they will accept patients whose primary health insurance is Medicaid?
4. Should doctors and other health providers be allowed to choose whether or not they will accept patients whose primary health insurance is Medicare?
5. How can we make health care more available in rural areas?

part three

HEALTHY LIFESTYLES

SERMON

thirteen · **GET MY PEOPLE GOING!!**

> *Blessed are those who hunger and thirst*
> *for righteousness, for they will be filled.*
>
> **Matthew 5:6**

Take your weight, and subtract 60 percent of it. That's what you really weigh—minus the water. We are all far lighter than we think!

Seriously, though, it's interesting to think how dependent and connected to water we are for life. Almost every function of our body depends on proper hydration.

The Institute of Medicine recommends that men consume about thirteen cups of water per day and women about nine cups of water per day. Even moderate dehydration can make us tired and less energetic. Dehydration can make one more susceptible to respiratory and urinary tract infections. And it can make one more likely to become, well, you know, um, *constipated*. And the older you get, the less likely you are to recognize that you are thirsty. Drinking enough water is a deep, basic, life-maintaining need.

It is perhaps, then, no accident that in Scripture we find passages about thirst—spiritual thirst—a deep, basic, life-maintaining need. In Matthew, chapter 5, we read, "Blessed are you who hunger and thirst for righteousness." The psalmist writes in Psalm 42:1–2a, "as the deer pants for flowing streams, so pants my soul for you O God. My soul thirsts for God" (ESV). In the Gospel of John, Jesus says, "Let anyone who is thirsty come to me, and let the one who believes in me drink" (John 7:37–38a).

Thirst. It's a driving force, a compelling force, a life-sustaining force. It motivates us far better than rules. We all are familiar with the Ten Commandments, which were shared by Moses for God's people in the wilderness.

There are other rules—lots of them! Like the "Health Commandments":

1. Thou shalt not leave the leave house without brushing your teeth.
2. Thou shalt not go to bed without brushing *and flossing* your teeth.
3. Thou shalt not eat so much dessert.
4. Thou shalt not let a day go by in which you, and your husband, and your children in your house, do not each get at least thirty minutes a day of vigorous exercise.
5. Thou shalt not lord it over anyone else if thou are young and vigorous, for verily, the days are coming, when you, too, will hit your middle age.
6. Thou shalt not eat only hamburgers and pizza but shall honor the lowly vegetables of the earth.
7. Thou shalt drink six to eight glasses of water a day, for no one can live on coffee alone.

They go on. But they aren't really very motivating, are they? And what are these rules for, anyway? They are intended to help keep us healthy, but to what end do we have our health?

The Pharisee who questioned Jesus knew his Ten Commandments. He knew the dietary laws. He knew the rules about cleanliness. He knew the ordinances about all the right ways to live, like "honor your father and your mother, so that you may live long in the land . . . your God is giving you." When the lawyer asked Jesus which law was greatest, Jesus summarized it like this:

"'You shall love . . . your God with all your heart, and with all your soul, and with all your mind.' This is the greatest and first commandment. And a second is like it: 'You shall love your neighbor as yourself.' On these two commandments hang all the law and the prophets" (Matt. 22:37–40).

The Pharisees are often portrayed as the bad guys in the Gospels. But in many ways, they really got it. They knew that there was no sense in following all these rules if they don't bring fullness of life. Life to you. Life to others.

What good is good health if you don't have something to live for? Something to care about, passionately? "You shall love . . . your God with all your heart, and all your soul, and with all your might," as stated in Deuteronomy 6:5, and "your neighbor as yourself."

So, what does this say about health? It says that health is not a solitary endeavor:

- brush your teeth,
- eat your turnips,
- get on your treadmill.

Health is, rather, about community: take care of yourself so that you can care passionately for others.

Let me tell you about someone who is passionate about health. It's Cathy White, a parish nurse at St. Margaret of Scotland. This Catholic parish is near botanical gardens. Recently Cathy invited folks to walk with her to Jerusalem. Not literally, of course—they would only be walking around their neighborhood. But, by combining their miles, she hoped they could walk the number of miles from their parish to Jerusalem during Lent.

Cathy hoped and prayed that fifty people would sign up. You know what? One hundred and sixty-five people signed up, including an eighty-six-year-old woman who walks fifteen miles each week. In the first three weeks, these Walkers to Jerusalem covered three thousand miles. Together they challenged each other, walked with each other, helped each another.

Jesus says, "Blessed are you, blessed are you, blessed are you." Not "thou shalt not, thou shalt not, thou shalt not." We are called *to* wholeness, *to* newness of life, *to* the wonder of love.

I could tell you that over 40 percent of American adults aged forty to seventy-four had prediabetes in 2000, and it's probably closer to half today. That data is from the U.S. Department of Health and Human Services and the National Institutes of Health. Not everybody with prediabetes develops diabetes, but many do. That should scare the soda out of us! Then I could tell you that exercise and changing one's diet can significantly reduce the risk of developing diabetes.

Perhaps, however, we are less motivated by guilt than by love. Perhaps we are called *to* our gardens. To our sidewalks. To our parks. To walk with, to *be* with, to *love* God and God's creation. To walk with, to be with, to love our neighbor. To be at home within ourselves, no matter who or where we are.

This is why I am inviting you today to participate in a new eight-week program called, "Get My People Going!!" This program invites each of us to choose three areas of our lives where we would like to cultivate growth. Maybe you want to walk more. Maybe I want help in remembering to drink more water. Maybe your husband wants to eat a healthier diet with more fruits and vegetables. Maybe your mother wants to spend more time with her friends. Maybe your neighbor longs to spend more time in prayer. This "invitation to wholeness" will offer us a chance to do just that. We can do it together.

God loves us, and invites us to use all our gifts—of heart, mind, soul, and strength—extravagantly. Each of us has been given unique and precious gifts: unique and precious minds, unique and precious bodies. We are called out by God, to walk, to run, to dance!

So come, all who hunger and thirst, come to the living water. Regardless of who we are, how we look, or what we have, God loves us all, and thirsts for our love. God has given us neighbors and thirsts for us to love them, too. Thirsts for us to walk with them, help them, care for them.

Let us not be bound by lassitude, anxiety, fear, or selfishness. Let us not live in regret for the past, but in hope for the morrow. We are invited to drink deeply at the springs of hope and compassion. We are called to come to the healing streams that refresh and make us whole.

So, friends, let us walk together, in this place, and in the world. Let us slowly learn how to pray and how to live. And let us ever remain close to the One who gives us beautiful lessons. Thanks be to God. Amen and amen.

SERMON

fourteen · **AND THEIR EYES WERE OPENED**

Then their eyes were opened, and they recognized him; and he vanished from their sight.

Luke 24:31a

In his wonderful book, *Surprises Around the Bend: 50 Adventurous Walkers*, Presbyterian minister Richard A. Hasler has gathered stories about fifty remarkable people who made walking an integral part of their creative process and wholistic living. He documents the work of transformative thinkers and leaders such as Dorothy Day, Mohandas Gandhi, Martin Luther King, Dietrich Bonhoeffer, Harriet Tubman, Thomas Merton, Emily Brontë, and others. Hasler shows how they built walking into their daily lives, and how that practice changed them physically, mentally, and spiritually.

Abraham Lincoln was one of those walkers profiled by Hasler. We all remember the story of how Lincoln walked a great distance to return a penny, right? But Hasler doesn't include this story. Certainly, he shares the description of Lincoln's walking style as penned by his law partner in Springfield, Illinois, William Herndon. Herndon writes about Lincoln:

> When he walked he moved cautiously but firmly; his arms and giant hands swung down by his side. He walked with an even tread, the inner sides of his feet being parallel. He put the whole foot flat down on the ground at once, not rising from the toe, and hence he had no spring to his walk. The whole man, body and mind, worked slowly, as if it needed oiling.[1]

Lincoln's pastor in Washington, D.C., Phineas Gurley, stated that Lincoln walked as if "he was about to plunge forward, from his right shoulder, for he always walked, when he had anything in his hand, as if he was pushing something in front of him."[2]

Despite his lack of form and grace, Lincoln walked with purpose. He walked when he was thinking things through, as he did in Springfield when he was contemplating asking Mary Todd to marry him. He walked when he was troubled, as he did in Washington during the war years from 1861 to 1865. Hasler writes, "Shocking those men who were pledged to protect him, he would frequently escape their watch and meander around the capital unarmed and seemingly afraid of no one."[3]

Lincoln also walked when he was seeking the good of those around him, as he did in 1865 in Richmond, Virginia, shortly before the war ended. One of his biographers writes,

> Jefferson Davis has already left the city, but many people remained in the city who were still hostile toward Lincoln. Instead of riding triumphantly through the fallen Southern capitol on a horse or in a carriage, Lincoln chose to walk the two miles from the dock into the heart of the city. He had with him his son and twelve sailors. He did not wait for the army offers who were supposed to guard him as he entered this hostile city. It was a quiet, solemn procession and he walked fearlessly as an astonished crowd lined the streets.[4]

Truly, exercise is not something all of us enjoy. Many of us share the sentiment of Mark Twain, who, on his seventieth birthday, stated, "I have never taken any exercise, except sleeping and resting, and I never intend to take any. Exercise is loathsome. And it cannot be any benefit when you are tired: and I was always tired. But let another person try my way, and see where he will come out."[5] It's no surprise that Mark Twain was not among those profiled in Hasler's book!

The very concept of *needing* exercise is a testament to the relative luxury in which we live our lives today. Nobody in Jesus's day had a car. Lives were hard—people were farmers, or fishermen, or carpenters. The women had much toil to feed, clothe, and raise a family. Few people then could afford any mode of transportation besides walking. Walking could be dangerous. Remember the story of the good Samaritan, who helped the man who was beaten and left for dead on the side of the road? So it was wise to have someone to accompany you, as the couple did on the road to Emmaus.

But what a surprise this couple got around the bend on their walk that day! They were walking from Jerusalem to Emmaus—probably their hometown. As they walked along, they talked together about all that had happened in Jerusalem recently. While they were talking, Jesus appeared and walked along with them, but "their eyes were kept from recognizing him." And Jesus said to them, "What are you discussing with each other while you walk along?" They stood still, looking sad. Then, one of them, whose name was Cleopas, answered him, "Are you the only stranger in Jerusalem, who does not know the things that have taken place these in these days?" Jesus asked them, "What things?" They replied, "The things about Jesus of Nazareth," and they went on to tell the whole story of his ministry, and his crucifixion, and what had happened at the tomb. As they came near Emmaus, Jesus walked ahead as if he were going on. But the couple urged him strongly, saying, "Stay with us, because it is almost evening and the day is now nearly over." So Jesus went in to stay with them. "When he was at the table with them, he took bread, blessed and broke it, and gave it to them. Then their eyes were opened, and they recognized him; and he vanished from their sight." (see Luke: 13–31).

This last part is the scripture that we remember, that we quote regularly during the order of worship for celebrating the sacrament of communion. But we should also remember the next verse: "That same hour they got up and returned [the seven miles back] to Jerusalem; and they found the eleven and their companions gathered together. . . . Then they told what had happened on the road, and how he had been made known to them in the breaking of the bread" (Luke 24:33–35).

You never know what surprise is around the bend for you if you put one foot in front of the other and step out the door. It may be a surprise in the form of new or renewed friendship as we share conversation with someone else on the journey. It may be a surprise in the form of renewed strength, as we find ourselves able to walk a little easier and a little further than the day before. Or it might be in finding God right there, with us, walking alongside, guiding our steps.

What can congregations do to promote walking and other forms of activity that are good for the body and the soul? Some congregations have introduced "Walking to Jerusalem," where you calculate the distance between your congregation and Jerusalem. In the case of the scripture we read today, that distance was only seven miles, but for most of the world's Christians, that distance is far greater. The program invites parishioners to sign up and try, by adding their miles together, to walk the distance between their home congregation and Jerusalem.

Some parishes have reprised that program for Advent as a "Walk to Bethlehem." Other churches have started weekly walking groups, or yoga classes, or tai chi, or armchair exercises. The joy in these groups is in the fellowship, and in the surprises around the bend. It is also in the deeper understanding we find in our own souls as we commune with God along the way.

Joyce Rupp is a Catholic sister in her early sixties, who at age sixty decided to walk the Camino pilgrimage in Spain with a friend. This journey of almost five hundred miles took over a month through fields, forests, cities, and a dry, hot, dusty plateau. She documents this physical and spiritual experience in her book, *Walk in a Relaxed Manner: Life Lessons from the Camino*. The title of her book is drawn from one of the most important lessons she learned during that time: to slow down. She writes,

> We soon discovered that the rushing and pushing caused us to lose our enjoyment of the walk itself. We left home in order to experience the freedom of *getting away from it all* but we simply took the tensions with us in new forms. The *place* of our stress changed but we had not changed. We continued to strain and groan under the desires and expectations of achievement and accomplishment—goals which our culture thrives on and implants in us almost from birth.[6]

By slowing down and savoring each day, her eyes were opened to recognize the newness of life that surrounded her:

> Gradually the Camino helped me see that every day is an adventure because every day is new. We have not lived that

day before. Every space of our lives is unknown until we live it. Approaching life in this way keeps it fresh, invigorating, alive, and inviting. There's something marvelous about stepping out each morning and touching new ground every step of the day. Each moment becomes an opening for revelation. Every footstep announces another opportunity for expansion of one's limited version and view of the world. How life-transforming it would be if each of us awakened to the new day with a sense of adventure in our hearts instead of a dread of work or a sluggish approach to what the day holds.[7]

So, let our eyes be opened to the surprises that lie around the bend for us as we step out in faith to embrace the opportunities ahead. We may face a day of desert wilderness, but springs of healing lie ahead. We may be walking toward a day of reconciliation like Lincoln faced, a day of transformation like Joyce Rupp experienced, or just a quiet walk home to Emmaus. But may we be open to the healing and transforming experiences of life as we remember that God walks with us. Thanks be to God! Amen.

REFLECTION

fifteen · **FINDING MAYO**

Therefore, since we are surrounded by so great a cloud of witnesses, let us also lay aside every weight and the sin that clings so closely, and let us run with perseverance the race that is set before us, looking to Jesus the pioneer and perfecter of our faith.

Hebrews 12:1-2a

Last night I took one of those Internet quizzes to "test your knowledge." This particular test was on the website www.Mayo Clinic.com (not to be confused with www.Mayo.com, which takes you to a food site, where I learned they now make mayonnaise with lime juice, too).

Anyway, this particular quiz was in the Senior Health Section of the Mayo Clinic site, and was entitled, "Aging Quiz: Secrets of Longevity." I wanted to know the secrets, or at least be assured that I already knew them.

The last question surprised me. It was, "What is the most common chronic ailment affecting seniors: arthritis, high blood pressure, or cardiovascular disease?" The answer was arthritis, but the statistics revealed some surprises in reverse: 42 percent of people over age seventy don't have arthritis, 55 percent don't have high blood pressure, and 79 percent don't have heart disease.

You may say, well, many of the people with heart disease died before they reached seventy, so that leaves the healthy, and you might be right. But these statistics point to the fact that many seniors stay remarkably well. Ninety-five percent of people over age sixty-five do not live in nursing homes, which is a good thing, since the average cost for a year in a U.S. nursing home is $40,000 per person.

Now it may be the fact that I just clicked over a big round number on my age odometer that is pushing me to ponder Paradise. But as the oh-so-youthful-looking Dr. Takahashi from Mayo Clinic points out, aging is not an event, it is a process that starts at birth. As baby boomers age, information about healthy aging can be found everywhere. For those who make healthy nutritional choices and exercise regularly, who stay connected to God and reach out to others, even if they have been dealt a chronic illness, the journey of aging can be eased. And in the meantime, grab the MayoLite, and keep moving! You're doing great!

REFLECTION

sixteen · **THEREFORE, CHOOSE LIFE**

*I have set before you life and death, blessings and curses.
Choose life so that you and your descendents
may live, loving the Lord your God.*

Deuteronomy 30:19b–20a

We, our country, and our world face serious choices about how we want to live and how we want to use our resources. Each of us, and we as a congregation, stand before our own unique set of choices about lifestyle and how our finite span of life, a sacred trust, might best honor and serve God.. Because we are people of faith, called to preach, teach, and heal, we believe there is more to our health promotion ministry than simply making prudent health investments in the community.

As Gary Gunderson and Larry Pray write in *The Leading Causes of Life*, "we need to act on the choices that lead to life, to extend ourselves in webs of blessing, and to nurture hope in all things . . . this is the way of life."[1] Which actions will we take today that will bring blessing, nurture hope, and forge community connections in meaningful ways?

Viktor Frankl, a psychotherapist who survived a concentration camp during the Holocaust, wrote in *Man's Search for Meaning*, "The meaning of our existence is not to be invented, but to be detected."[2] We are not here today to invent God's will for our choices, but to seek God's will.

We plant the seed; God waters. Does it matter what we grow, if this harvest feeds, restores, and blesses the children and their families, and brings helps to support the leading causes of life such as increased agency to act on one's own behalf and on behalf of others, stronger connection to the wider community, location of meaningful vocation, wholistic health, and brighter hope for tomorrow?

God spoke a word to the young prophet Jeremiah when the people of Israel were in exile in Babylon, asking him to share this message of hope with his people: "For surely I know the plans I have for you, says God, plans for your welfare and not for harm, to give you a future and a hope" (Jer. 29:11).

Addressing this list of needs for health and wholeness is not an easy task! It is not about a lack of will on the part of those who would do good. Reinhold Niebuhr, writing about choices at an earlier time in U.S. history, noted that "no group of idealists can easily move the pattern of history toward the desired goal of peace and justice. The recalcitrant forces in the historical drama have a power and persistence beyond our reckoning."[3]

There are many forces acting on children and families today, and the needs are positively overwhelming. The actions congregations take today will not eliminate poverty, keep every child from homelessness, teach every child to read, find every child a primary care physician, or keep every child healthy and whole. Yet, still, can we do other?

Let us rejoice in the tremendous opportunity and privilege it is to contribute to the common good, following in the footsteps of God's people in every time and age, people who have elected to act on behalf of the "least of these." In this day, in this time, all choices that improve the lot of those in need of help are good ones.

REFLECTION

seventeen · **MANNA: WHEN ENOUGH IS ENOUGH**

> *Then God said to Moses, "I am going to rain bread from heaven for you, and each day the people shall go out and gather enough for that day. In that way I will test them, whether they will follow my instructions or not. On the sixth day, when they prepare what they bring in, it will be twice as much as they gather on other days."*
>
> **Exodus 16:4–5**

The Bible says some rather strange things, in the context of today's world. When the people of Israel found manna in the wilderness, Moses told them, "Each one is to gather as much as he needs. No one is to keep any of it until morning." Hoarders found leftovers reeking and full of maggots. On the eve of the Sabbath, Moses told people to save what was left and keep it until morning. Those who did not discovered there was no manna to be found on the day of rest.

In our day and age, we all want to be sure we have enough of everything for today and for our future. So, how much is "enough?" If we are talking about trans fats, even a few grams a day are bad for you. What about exercise? New guidelines say thirty minutes daily is best to maintain weight, sixty minutes a day for weight loss. Sleep—eight hours a night (more than 60 percent of adults sleep fewer hours, the National Sleep Foundation reports), but not more than nine, for too much sleep increases your heart attack risk. Sex—depends on whom you ask!

Water—six to eight glasses a day. Wine—one glass of red wine a day, if at all. Fruits and vegetables—five to nine servings a day. Bread, meat, dairy products—the list goes on.

What about health care? How much screening is enough for cancer? For depression? For HIV/AIDS? In the treatment of illness, which drug is the right one, and how much, how long? Health professionals often differ on deciding what is "enough."

Then there is our social health: How many hours each week should we be working? How much should we relax with our family? How much time should we pray? How many hours should our kids watch TV? How much time should we spend with our friends?

And what about our "stuff"? How many square feet do we need in our home? How much land do we need for our lawn? How many malls do we need in a town? How much money and possessions are enough for us to be truly whole? How do we find a balance that brings health?

What is enough? It's a healthy question for clergy and parish nurses to ask of themselves and their congregations.

REFLECTION

eighteen · **WE DO NOT LIVE BY STRESS ALONE**

> *Then Jesus was led up by the Spirit into the wilderness to be tempted by the devil. He fasted forty days and forty nights, and afterwards he was famished. The tempter came and said to him, "If you are the Son of God, command these stones to become loaves of bread." But Jesus answered, "One does not live by bread alone, but by every word that comes from the mouth of God."*
>
> **Matthew 4:1–4**

T*he Washington Post* recently reported that baby boomers appear to be less healthy than their parents were at the same age. Researchers from the University of Texas at Austin found that "the trend seems to be that people are not as healthy as they approach retirement as they were in older generations." The study reports that "boomers tend to report more stress than earlier generations— from their jobs, their commutes, taking care of their parents and their kids—all of which can take a physical toll, which is compounded by having less support from extended families and communities."[1]

Lisa Berkman of the Harvard School of Public Health says, "People are working two jobs. They are not sleeping as much. They're experiencing more job insecurity. They have less time to take care of themselves. They are more socially isolated."[2]

Thirty-two years ago, German theologian Dorothee Sölle published a book about the "inner journey," considering religious experiences, texts, and their interpretations. Translated later under the title *Death by Bread Alone*, Sölle discussed our need for liberation. Like Jesus, who, when tempted, replied, "Man does not live by bread alone," she reminds us that true life lies in finding meaning and purpose, having compassion for those who are suffering, and creating a sense of community with others.

Parish nurses and health ministers have a tremendous opportunity to make a difference in today's world. They see the strain of people taking care of aging parents and children with special needs. They hear the stress of people who work full-time but do not have health insurance for themselves, yet earn too much for their children to be eligible. They know the anxiety of people who struggle with chronic illness. They reach out to people who are longing for meaning, for connection, for hope.

Recently, I heard a statistic that 80 percent of twenty-year-olds in the United States have never been to church (other than to a wedding or funeral). I'm assuming they are not adherents of other faiths, either. What spiritual hope are we offering them?

Integrating spirituality and health has been the mission of faith communities for millennia. Finding new ways to make that possible to all generations within changing societies is always a challenge. Congregations are uniquely poised to offer a vision of community and healing that can offer sustenance and hope to all.

HEALTHY LIFESTYLES
Discussion Questions

1. How might the church play a role in promoting healthy lifestyles?
2. In which areas of our church's life could we make changes to promote healthy lifestyles?
3. Who in our congregation might become a leader in helping us promote healthy lifestyles?
4. What opportunities are there for us to connect with the community in promoting healthy lifestyles?
5. How can we recognize efforts in this congregation to promote healthy lifestyles?

part four

HEALTHY FAMILIES

SERMON

nineteen · **SUFFER THE CHILDREN**

> *Suffer the children to come unto me,*
> *and forbid them not,*
> *for of such is the reign of God.*
>
> **Luke 18:16 (YLT)**

Zhou Jiaying, or "Bella," is a ten-year-old girl in Shanghai, China. Like most of the children her age in China, she is an only child. Like many other urban children her age in China, Bella is busy. Her weekly schedule has included classes in English, acting, piano, and swimming. After school she does homework until her parents come home, then it is time to practice the piano, and the only TV program she is permitted to watch is the news. Saturdays she takes a private essay class and then goes to Math Olympics. Sundays are for piano lessons and taking a prep class for an entrance exam. The entrance exam is to a middle school. She has a little time to stop for a Popsicle before heading home to do homework on Friday afternoon, when school lets out early.

Why are Bella's parents keeping her so busy? "We don't want to be brutal to her," says Bella's father. "But in China, the environment doesn't let you do anything else."

When told that children in America do not often do homework on Friday afternoons, Bella sighed and said, "They must be very happy."[1]

Ellin is an eleven-year-old girl who lives with her mother in New Zealand. She is from South Korea, where her dad works as an ophthalmologist. More than four years ago, her mother took her and her brother abroad to study English, and they seldom see their father. About forty thousand school-aged South Korean kids are studying abroad.

Her mother, Park Jeong-won, said that "she talked to her husband a couple of hours daily by phone . . . [but that] her son and daughter never asked to talk to their father. He, in turn, never asked to talk to his children.

"Asked whether she missed her father, Ellin said: 'I don't miss him that much. I see him every year.'"[2]

It's a relief to know that children in America generally don't have to work so hard or live so far away from a parent. But they are busy, too, with growing amounts of homework starting in kindergarten. With preparation for ever more standardized tests. With music lessons. Sports practices. American children are overscheduled too. Some are finding healthy ways to relax. But far too many turn to tobacco, drugs, or alcohol.

Results from a substance abuse screening test administered by Dr. John Knight and colleagues at Harvard Medical School and Boston Children's Hospital indicate that "[a]bout 80 percent of teens have begun to drink and half have used an illegal drug by senior year in high school. 'Substance use is associated with the leading causes of death among U.S. teenagers: unintentional injuries, homicides and suicides.' Depression, conduct disorder and unplanned sexual activity are also associated with substance use."[3]

A few years ago, the National Center on Addiction and Substance Abuse at Columbia University in New York launched a new initiative called "Family Day: A Day to Eat Dinner with Your Children."™ They even trademarked the name. Research by the National Center on Addiction and Substance Abuse (CASA) at Columbia University consistently found that the more often children eat dinner with their families, the less likely they are to smoke, drink, or use drugs. They found that "compared to kids who have fewer than three family dinners per week, children and teens who have frequent family dinners are at 70% lower risk for substance abuse; one-third less likely to try alcohol, half as likely to try cigarettes or marijuana, and half as likely to get drunk monthly."[4] This time for relaxation and relationship-building with family is hugely important to kids of all ages.

We know that this is not easy. Most jobs don't end until 5:00 P.M., and for most who work outside the home there are errands and a commute before dinner can be started. Most of us no longer live in farm families in remote areas. I was lucky during my own childhood in rural Alberta, where the school bus dropped us off at 4:00 in the afternoon and there we stayed until the bus picked us up the next morning (save the weekly piano lesson Saturday and the trip to town on Saturday, or the rare—and I do mean rare—school event or visit to a friends' house).

But isn't there some happy medium for our overprogrammed, overstressed kids, and some way that families can reclaim some time together?

It's not around the TV set. According to the Nielson rating people, the average school child spends 900 hours per year in school, and 1500 hours per year watching television. Fifty-four percent of children surveyed would rather watch TV than spend time with their parents anyway. And this doesn't even count the time spent on video and computer games or doing various things on the phone.

Jesus said, "Suffer the little children to come unto me, and forbid them not, for of such is the reign of God." So, just what is it in the reign of God that the children have access to?

Time. Plenty of time. They have the rest of their lives. It is we adults who think that everything must be "hurry up and wait." How many times did you ask your kids to hurry up this week?

Joy. On one of his annual joke shows, Garrison Keillor, the host of Prairie Home Companion, claimed children laugh a couple of hundred times a day, while adults laugh fewer than a couple of dozen times.

Energy. How often do we tell the kids, "Don't run in the house, don't run in the halls, don't run in church"?

Trust. We're the ones telling kids not to talk to strangers. They would talk to adults if left to their own devices.

Hope. Childhood is that time of life when all kids believe it is possible to be president, or a doctor, or a movie star. All things are possible to those who believe.

No wonder Jesus told the disciples to back off, and to observe. The children were bringing healthy minds, bodies, and spirits. The adults were the ones who were so tightly scheduled—in first-century Palestine, no less—that there was no room for the joy, energy, trust, or hope of the children. Just think of the hope of that little guy who brought the two loaves and the fishes. What a meal! What a family day that must have been!! What child would have wanted to sniff glue or smoke a joint that day? What parents would have worried that their child needed to work harder, harder, harder to get ahead in the presence of Jesus?

This is not a sermon opposing homework or music or sports. It is simply a call to balance in all of our lives—for children and adults. Yes, life is hard. It is competitive and there are many trials—from the rising cost of gas to worry about getting into college (and paying for it). But we cannot sacrifice our children on the altar of our stress. They are children we need to nurture and protect. And we are all part of the family of God, who will show us the way.

SERMON

twenty · THE WISDOM OF ELDERS

> *Happy are those who find wisdom, and those who get understanding, for her income is better than silver, and her revenue better than gold. She is more precious than jewels, and nothing you desire can compare with her. Long life is in her right hand; in her left hand are riches and honor. Her ways are ways of pleasantness and all her paths are peace. She is a tree of life to those who lay hold of her; those who hold her fast are called happy.*
>
> **Proverbs 3:13–18**

Not long ago, I was in a university library trying to copy an article for a research project. I say "trying to copy" because I was having a little trouble figuring out the photocopying machine. I am used to the copy machine in our parish nurse office. I can figure out the copy machine in the church office. But this one was different.

First, you put money into a machine to encode a card with a dollar's worth of copies. Then you pushed a button to get the card back. Then you put it into a different slot to add more copies. When you've loaded it up with enough money, you're finally ready to tackle the copier.

Now, this particular copier resembled a farm implement more than an office machine. It was huge, coming up to about my chest. Somewhere on that machine should have been a slot for my copy card. I looked up one side and down the other without luck. Finally, I asked a young university student near me where to put the card. She looked at me like I was brain dead, and pointed to a place beside me. I needed to put my card into a third machine to activate the copier.

Well, I made my copies and scurried off. What I really wanted to do, though, was scold that girl. "Just you wait, young lady," I wanted to say. "The years will fly by and soon you'll be older than fifty, asking for help. Or you'll be elderly, longing to be seen as a woman and not just old." But what could I really say? The world tells her everywhere that youth and health is what life is all about.

The world would have us all believe that life is for the lucky and the strong. For the young and the restless. For the rich and powerful. For the healthy, the married, the employed, the person of the right race and gender. But the Bible turns that worldly wisdom on its head. It is filled with stories of people of all ages, caring about one another. It is filled with tales of people who weren't famous. Not rich, nor powerful, nor always healthy. But loved. Loved by God. The Bible is filled with hope for persons like you and I.

Remember the story of Naomi in the Old Testament? Naomi was a woman whose adult sons and husband had died. She was left with two foreign-born daughters-in-law, and she wanted to leave Moab and return to Israel, the land of her birth. One daughter-in-law returned to her own family, but Ruth, who was from Moab, insisted on going with Naomi. "Where you go, I'll go. Where you stay, I'll stay. Your people shall be my people. Your God shall be my God" (Ruth 1:16).

Ruth's compassion for her mother-in-law led her to a new land and to a new life. Ruth's kindness led her to Boaz, who became her husband, and they became the ancestors of King David. But the beauty of this story is in the way that these two women cared for one another, when they had nothing—gleaning for grain in the fields for their daily bread.

Didn't look like much of an investment, this investment of time and effort in caring about an older woman. But there was a lot of wisdom here. There was the wisdom of Naomi who knew that, for herself, she needed to return to her homeland. She also was wise enough not to force her daughters-in-law to come with her. There was also the wisdom of Ruth, who found that the ways of peace and pleasantness are indeed honorable ways, leading to the tree of life.

Currently, there are 37.2 million seniors who live in the United States. Many of them are very healthy, but all of them will die, as will we. They might die from an accident, a short illness, or a traumatic event, like a heart attack. More likely they will die following an illness that progresses rather slowly over a couple of years.

Who will care for the sick elderly? Primarily, their families will. According to the U.S. Department of Health and Human Services, the typical family caregiver is a forty-six-year-old woman caring for her widowed mother. Most of those caregivers are employed, and more than half of them have to make adjustments to their work—either working fewer hours, going in late, or quitting altogether. How can we honor the elderly *and* support their families in their compassion and their giving of care?

There are many ways in which the church can make a difference. The Volunteer Interfaith Caregiving Program of the Robert Wood Johnson Foundation has helped many congregations work together to provide assistance to caregivers and families around the nation. The Stephen's Ministry Program is also a great assistance to families needing support, and many congregations work closely with hospice, as well.

Having a parish nurse available is a huge help to many families who are caring for elderly parents, particularly if there is distance involved. One middle-aged woman, Nancy, whose father was helped by a parish nurse writes,

> I know my Dad feels enormously grateful for Ellen's help and attention, but I feel that I benefited the most! It's difficult to be fifteen hundred miles away when your sole surviving parent is ailing. I don't recall how Ellen's name came to me, but I telephoned her after my father returned home from surgery. She visited him and was my salvation a few days later when he began having chest pains. One phone call from me, and Ellen picked him up and drove him to the hospital, waiting with him in the ER while tests were run and evaluated—a five-hour ordeal! Ellen was the "health care professional" member of our small, family-based "team" with whom I communicated by e-mail during my Dad's tribulations. His heretofore unknown "parish nurse" lent her considerable strength and attention to us during what turned out to be a three-month road to recovery. Ellen visited my father often. . . . She genially but perceptively listened to his complaints, queried his doctors, and shared her observations about him with me on the phone

and by e-mail. She answered millions of little questions doctors don't have time for, but whose answers make a lot of difference to patients. She was invaluable in sharing resources as I built a list of caregivers and services and advised me well on navigating the insurance system. She reminded me of my Dad's important patient rights, and I found creative ways to keep everyone in the loop. The comfort I felt knowing Ellen was there if my Dad needed her was enormous.[1]

This is the ministry of the church—to care for widows—and widowers!—and orphans in their need. To heal the sick, feed the hungry, clothe the naked, visit those who are in prison. To accompany those who are on a journey home.

We find wisdom as we listen to our elders and find out where they want to go, what they want to do. They may not want aggressive medical treatment for a progressive condition. And then again, they might. They need to play the primary role in their own care, as much as they are able.

We also find wisdom as we listen to our own hearts and respond with compassion to their needs, as well as ours. We find wisdom as we share our burdens with others. We find wisdom as we seek diligently after God's ways.

I must admit that I was, like the girl at the copier, a young, impatient college girl. I looked at thirty-year-olds like they should have their birthdays announced by Willard Scott on "Today." But I thank God for a little wisdom that aging brings. I thank God for each wonderful day of life, and for health. I thank God for the church, which rallies around the lost and the lone, the hungry and the sick. And I thank God for all those who respond with wisdom and grace to the needs of others. God bless you, now and always. Amen and amen.

REFLECTION

twenty-one · LORD, HELP US!

But she came and knelt before him, saying, "Lord, help me."
Matthew 15:25

I am a clergyperson working in health ministry. I am also the wife of a seminary professor and the mother of two children. The latter is my most challenging role! One of our children is autistic, and I have observed through personal experience, through working with other professionals, and through talking with other parents of children with autism that the special challenges presented by children on the autism spectrum present unique opportunities for pastoral care.

There are many different types of mental health challenges faced by families today, families you will find in every congregation. These mental health challenges can range from cognitive developmental disabilities to mental disorders to mental illnesses. The National Institute on Disability and Rehabilitation Research compiles data on the prevalence of mental health concerns, some of which are included here:

> ***Mental retardation:*** About 2.5 million noninstitutionalized people have mental retardation. Approximately 700,000 other people with mental retardation are living in institutional settings.
>
> ***Mental disorders:*** 28.1 percent of Americans (51.3 million) have a mental disorder in any given one-year period. About 2.8 percent of the adult population (five million) experience severe mental disorders in a one-year period.

Mental illness: 1.8% (3.3 million people) have a serious mental illness.[1]

For the purposes of this discussion, I would like to focus on one type of mental health concern—ministry to parents of children with autism—to open discussion on the topic of mental health issues in congregations.

The prevalence of autism is growing rapidly in this country. There has been a 20 percent annual growth in the incidence (diagnosis of new cases) of autism over the past decade. The Center for Disease Control and Prevention's (CDC's) Autism and Developmental Disabilities Monitoring Network found that in 2007 about one out of every 150 eight-year-old children in the United States had an autism spectrum disorder (ASD).

The National Institute of Mental Health states that children with an ASD "demonstrate (1) deficits in social interaction, (2) deficits in verbal and nonverbal communication, and (3) repetitive behaviors or interests. In addition, they will often have unusual responses to sensory experiences, such as to certain sounds or to the way objects look. Each of these symptoms runs the gamut from mild to severe and will present in each individual child differently."[2] Another child is diagnosed with an ASD every minute in this country.

Karen Siff Exkorn, parent of a child with autism and the author of *The Autism Sourcebook*, writes: "I desperately needed advice on how to cope with my own personal and emotional issues. It seemed nearly impossible to maintain hope for our son, who had a condition for which there was said to be no cure. So I found myself on an emotional roller coaster of denial, acceptance, and pure rage—and I couldn't figure out a way to stop it."[3]

Most clergy and health ministers are likely to run across parents of children with autism. I would like to explore from a pastoral perspective some of the concerns that may be held by these parents, and to suggest ten ideas for working with this population of adults.

1. Autism is a fearsome diagnosis for parents, even if it is a relief to know what is going on. *Listen to their fears.* Parents of children with autism can be harboring fears regarding a number of

issues. They may fear that their children will not be able to learn the basics needed to survive in the world today. They may worry that their child will not be able to attend regular school or to develop friendships. They may be anxious that their child will not be able to support him- or herself through employment as an adult, or that their child might, at some point in life, experience physical or sexual abuse at the hands of others. Parents also may fear that their children might fall victim to bullies or scams. Or they may worry that, despite their best efforts, they won't be able to leave a large enough financial legacy to support their autistic son or daughter throughout adulthood. The list goes on: where will these children live, how will they pay their bills, will they be able to marry, to have children of their own, and take care of them if they do?

Clergy and health ministers are safe people for these parents—a comfort as a nonjudgmental ear. Your listening is an incredible blessing and help. Their concerns are valid and real.

2. There is more to their child than simply the autistic spectrum disorder. *Listen to the joys.* Every child has positive attributes, whether it is physical beauty, the joy of the occasional hug, the wonder of his or her strength and determination, or the progress the child is making along the way. *Encourage the parents to talk about what they love about their child—often.*

3. *Encourage the parents to rest.* Sleep disorders are high among children with autism, and it can be years before the parents learn that this is typical. Help them to identify ways to provide safety for their child and still get sleep themselves.

4. *Encourage them to make time for intimacy with their partner.* Having a child with special needs is very hard on marriages, and having a child with autism can be a profound stress on a relationship. The divorce rate among parents of children with autism is high—some sources say as high as 80 percent. In 2007, the National Autism Association launched a national divorce study for parents of autistic children, and the results of that study are pending. A wonderful book to which you might refer parents is *Married with Special Needs Children:*

A Couples' Guide to Keeping Connected by Laura Marshak and Fran Prezant.

5. *Help parents to work on the issue of control.* Reinhold Niebuhr's "Serenity Prayer" was called the "Courage Prayer" by one of his biographers, because she believed that Niebuhr meant we needed to have the courage to change the things we could, and the wisdom to know over what we needed to give up control, and then have the serenity to accept those things we couldn't change. There is much that parents of children with autism can do! Early interventions such as Applied Behavioral Analysis (ABA), Relationship Development Intervention (RDI), speech therapy, and sensory diets as part of occupational therapy often can have a profound positive effect. Staying proactive for one's children is a lifelong task. But still, there comes that point where one must have serenity about those things that truly cannot be changed. Helping parents struggle with finding that wisdom is a huge gift.

6. *Help parents identify anger management strategies for themselves and their other children.* Children with autism often get stuck—they perseverate—in self-comforting or "self-stimming" (self-stimulating) behaviors that are atypical at best and asocial at worst. These behaviors can include obsessively dropping pencils or rocks, constantly pouring water, rocking, or sexually stimulating oneself in inappropriate settings. Parents want kids to stop these actions, and often with intervention (and sometimes without) these behaviors do diminish. In the meantime, however, the parents are going mad watching this action happen over and over for no good reason that they can see.

These behaviors can also be annoying for siblings, who request that the parent make the autistic brother or sister stop the actions in question, because they know that they themselves could never get away with such activity. It seems hypercritical to them for a parent to "let" it continue, and yet that sibling (generally) understands that his or her brother or sister has autism and often is mad at the disorder, too. Aargh! This can happen often enough during one day—let alone a whole lifetime—to make anyone feel insane (but it is amazing to what the human spirit can adjust). Anger management strategies are a good thing—for the whole family!

7. It is isolating to have children with an ASD—who wants to invite this family over for dinner? *Help the parents identify a circle of support for themselves,* making friends through hobbies, connecting with fellow members of their faith communities, or attending support groups for parents of special needs children. No one quite understands the life of a parent with an autistic child as well as another parent facing a similar family situation.

8. It is also worrisome to wonder if your child can develop friendships. *Encourage the parents to talk with their child's teacher and school counselor about this concern.* Often school counselors or social workers can help to develop a "Circle of Friends" for special-needs children. These can be formed anytime from the early elementary grades through high school.

9. Years ago, parents of children with autism (particularly mothers) were blamed for being "cold" and "causing" the autism. *Help parents remember that the autism is not their fault:* they did not purposely cause autism to come upon their child by any of their actions. Connecting with other parents of children with autism can help to address this. There are often local support groups or parents can connect with one online through a resource such as www.autismspeaks.org.

10. *Finally, remind them that God will not leave them (or their child) alone.* Even severe autism cannot separate a child or an adult from the love of God. A full and rich spiritual life is still possible for them and for their child. Mostly, what you can do for parents of children living with autism is to love and support them. Their lives will have tremendous ups and downs, and challenges for many years ahead. Sometimes it is one day at a time, and often it is one minute at a time. Being a listening and supportive ear may make all the difference in the world for these families.

Now, having said all this about autism, the same is true for *any* family facing *any* mental health issues: they need our unconditional love and support, they need our listening ears, and they need our acceptance and welcome.

Perhaps Howard J. Clinebell Jr., said it best in his groundbreaking classic, *The Mental Health Ministry of the Local Church*.

1. Mental health is a central and inescapable concern of any local church that is a healing-redemptive fellowship.
2. A local church today has an unprecedented opportunity to multiply its contributions to both the preventative and the therapeutic dimensions of mental health.
3. A church can seize this opportunity most effectively by allowing mental health to become a leavening concern, permeating all areas of its life. When this occurs, the spirit of Christian community flourishes in the many facets of a church's program, causing it to become a center of healing and growth.[4]

May it be so, Lord. Help us all!

REFLECTION

twenty-two · **IDENTIFIED: FLYING TOILETS**

> *I am about to do a new thing;*
> *now it springs forth, do you not perceive it?*
> *I will make a way in the wilderness*
> *and rivers in the desert.*
>
> Isaiah 43:19

Recently, *The New York Times* ran an article on public health in the developing world that stated that each year more than two million children die of diarrhea and other illnesses related to "lack of access to sanitation." An astounding 2.6 billion people—more than *one-third* of the world's population—have no toilets. More than a billion—one in six—drink water polluted by feces. The article referred to "flying toilets," which are plastic bags used for excrement and then tossed into the street.[1]

At first glance, this has little to do with most of us in America, including those in most congregations. Almost all of us in this country live in places where toilets and clean drinking water are taken for granted.

Yet this *is* related to the people who are in congregations, particularly congregations who are interested in outreach and those who have parish nurses. The more parish nurses I meet, the more I see their mission focus and interest in reaching out to others, even on the other side of the globe.

In a recent study I did of a small group of long-term parish nurses, I found that two-thirds had traveled abroad at some time related to their parish nursing work, either to explore the relationship between faith and health in another country, or to work with a health-related mission project.

Parish nursing is growing rapidly in many places—and along with it, partnerships of care between communities, sometimes separated by thousands of miles. There is growing interest in working together, joining hands with others around the world.

I believe that God is calling us to do a new thing in our own cities and towns and in partnership with those at home and abroad. I am grateful for the many passionate, globally minded parish nurses I meet who continue to raise the bar for caring for neighbors.

It's a small world, and it's getting smaller all the time. Thanks be to God for the opportunity to participate in this remarkable movement of the Spirit.

REFLECTION

twenty-three · GETTING OUT OF THE HOUSE

> *That same day Jesus went out of the house and sat beside the lake.*
>
> **Matthew 13:1**

I know a woman who works full-time in ministry, is married to another church professional, and has two kids, both of whom have special needs. Her parents and inlaws have challenging health concerns, ranging from neurodegenerative diseases to cardiovascular conditions, to increasing dementia. She is not unusual. I know, because I'm that woman, and I see plenty of others like me.

Those who are in the ministry are often also caring for aging parents, children of various ages (including grown children, which brings its own set of challenges for parenting!), while trying to pursue professional and personal goals. Most clergy are compensated (albeit at a modest scale compared to most professionals). Fewer parish nurses are paid for their health ministry: many are compensated on a part-time basis, and a great many others contribute their ministry without pay. A worker in God's vineyard can feel squeezed and eaten alive—the proverbial "sandwich!"

Add to that mix the very nature of the work of clergy and others in ministry, including parish nurses: they are caring for an unpredictable number of parishioners, congregational neighbors, and others in the community, caring for people in the context of family, from birth through death, in sickness and in health, for richer, for poorer . . . you get the picture. It is a recipe for a rich, creative ministry, and also a recipe for burnout.

Who is caring for the leaders of the church?

It takes courage to be a clergyperson or a parish nurse. You don't have a hospital floor and assigned patients—you have an entire congregation and the entourage that comes along with them—the neighborhood, relatives, the wider community (and the other staff!)

It takes dedication to be a clergyperson or a parish nurse. You must be constantly inventing programming, learning about resources, updating your knowledge bank, meeting new people, and being a daily self-starter.

All this you do in the context of your own needs. You may have served a congregation for a number of years and be wondering what might be in store for you next in your career. You may be facing family challenges, or your own physical, mental, or spiritual health issues. You may just need a break, a renewal, a new spiritual practice.

Who is caring for you?

First of all, it is important to remember that God is caring for you. There are people who want to help you—reach out and let them help with this work. Take time to sit or walk in prayer with God, who will guide you through to make the choices that need to be made in your ministry. You will find the way through to places of healing and wholeness. And give thanks, for you are doing this work because of your conviction that it is what God wants in your life, and that it is a way to make a difference in the life of a faith community.

Second, it is important to remember that you will never be able to do it all. And remember that you are never behind! No matter where you are in your work, if you are helping someone, then you are on time and doing the right thing.

Finally, remember that health ministry is a ministry of the entire church, not just of church leaders. All the gifts and talents of the body of Christ are needed to work together for healing and wholeness, including the healing and wholeness of the clergy, the parish nurses, the health cabinet, and all who are involved in the healing ministries of the congregation. Draw on the help of the entire church.

REFLECTION

twenty-four · NO PAIN, NO GAIN

> *Where there is no vision,*
> *the people perish . . .*
>
> **Proverbs 29:18a KJV**

Today, it seems like everywhere you turn, you are being bombarded with health information, from supermarket bulletin boards to signs on the inside of bathroom stalls. Having health information available is good, very good indeed. I *want* to know that germs cause disease and not be held in thrall by superstitions that posit that disease is caused by angry gods. I *want* to know that drinking lots of water may help avoid a recurrence of kidney stones so that I can do something about it. I *want* to know that eating lots of leafy green vegetables helps to protect the health of one's eyes.

But beyond health information, what really would help me is inspiration and hope to keep on keeping on with healthy practices. To be perfectly honest, what would help me many days is inspiration and hope to get out of bed and face the day.

We are all going to die, no matter how much health information we have. My parents are going to die, my siblings are going to die, I am going to die, my children are going to die. You are going to die. The entire human race will eventually be gone from the planet. So the hope is for a better life today, next year, ten years from now, as well as leaving a healthy planet for future generations.

With this in mind, I suggest the "PAIN" model for health, which I outline below.

Prudence. This is just the basic, good common sense stuff about health. Eat five to nine servings of vegetables and fruits every day. Get eight hours of sleep per night. Find a way to fit in thirty minutes of exercise a day (which means you have to give up thirty minutes of something else—there is no other way). Don't smoke or use drugs. Wear your seatbelt. Limit your alcohol intake. Limit your intake of deli meats with nitrates. Don't eat so much salt. Take a multivitamin that is appropriate for your age and health situation. Drink six to eight glasses of water a day. Pray. Keep a sense of humor. And remember: all things in moderation, including moderation.

Acceptance. You're not as young as you used to be. You can't live on coffee. You need to sleep sometime. You have to live with the genes you were dealt. Use it or lose it. If you have a chronic health condition, you have to take care of yourself. The market goes down as well as up. We all die. But don't forget that acceptance also means positive things: God loves us all—no exceptions. Accept that God really, truly loves you. Accept the reality of hope, kindness, and compassion in the world.

Individuality. Everybody is unique. You may be one of those rare people who smokes two packs of cigarettes a day and lives to be ninety-eight (but you probably aren't). Or you may be one of those rare people who gets breast cancer in her thirties (but you probably aren't). Your body is unique, and so is your health situation. Treat yourself with kindness and love, err on the side of caution in health practices, and know that you are beloved of God.

Needs. Honor your needs—you *need* exercise—even if you don't want it. You *need* sleep—even if you want to stay up and watch your favorite late-night show on TV. You *need* fruits and vegetables—even if you just want to have a piece of toast and a cup of tea. You *need* purpose and meaning in your life—even if the regular paycheck of your current job seems like it alone should fulfill you. You need God. You need prayer. Without vision, people perish.

PAIN—Prudence, acceptance, individuality, and needs. No PAIN, no gain!

HEALTHY FAMILIES
Discussion Questions

1. How does our congregation support the wholistic health of children?
2. How does our congregation build bridges between the generations?
3. How does our congregation support the needs of the "sandwich generation?"
4. How does our congregation care for caregivers?
5. How does our congregation model a healthy response to consumerism and its effects on families?

part five

HEALING OUR INFIRMITIES

SERMON

twenty-five · **LISTENING FOR THE SHEER SILENCE**

> *And after the earthquake a fire,*
> *but God was not in the fire; and after the fire*
> *a sound of sheer silence.*
>
> I Kings 19:12

A few days ago, I took my husband to the airport. Our two eleven-year-olds and I were taking him there to catch a flight to Israel for a few days. My husband teaches at Eden Seminary and travels a fair amount. I often drive him to the airport because we are too frugal—OK, cheap—to pay for a taxi or the parking garage. So we know the route well—up Brentwood, up 170, over to the airport, back on 70, back down 170, onto Brentwood, home.

But it was not that easy last Tuesday. My husband, as I said, travels a fair amount. What that means is that he always wants to leave at the very last minute so that he doesn't have to spend any more time than necessary in the airport. What that also means is that I go stark raving mad each time he travels worrying that something will come up and he will miss his flight.

Well, on this particular day, something came up. They were working on the intersection of Highway 170 and Brentwood Boulevard. And on this particular day, they had all the lanes trying to head northbound onto 170, all merging into one lane right there. And the cars going onto those lanes were coming from the north, and the south, and the east and the west.

At that point, as a transplant from Canada, living with my South Dakotan husband, I was wondering why we weren't living in a little house on the prairie. What were we doing here??

Life in the city, life in the twenty-first century, almost makes one long for a simpler time, before interstates, airports, cell phones, e-mail, and blogs. It makes one long for the simple pleasures of life.

Yet our scripture readings today remind us that life has never really been easy for people of any age. Elijah the prophet was afraid for his life when he challenged the murderous actions of Queen Jezebel and her husband, King Ahab of Samaria. He was afraid that he, too, would die, so he fled to the wilderness. Yet, God did not leave him alone. He was hungry, and God fed him cake—cake!—baked on hot stones, and gave him a jar of water to drink. He traveled to a cave, where he hid in despair.

Again, God did not leave the prophet alone. God came to Elijah, but not in the strong wind that split the mountains and rocks in pieces. God came to him, but not in the earthquake that shook the earth. God came to him, but not in the fire that blazed around the rock.

God came to Elijah in the sound of sheer silence. When Elijah heard the silence, he wrapped his face in his coat and went out and stood at the entrance of cave. Then there came a voice to him that asked, "What are you doing here, Elijah?"

What are you doing here, Elijah? What are you doing here? What are YOU doing here? This is a question that God asks each of us, in the silence of our own wilderness journeys.

Our wilderness journeys may lead us many places. They may lead us to other neighborhoods. They may lead us to other jobs. They may lead us to other destinations than the ones for which we set out. Sometimes there are amazing surprises and joy. Sometimes there are challenges and setbacks we did not anticipate.

Our wilderness journeys may lead us into a short illness or a chronic disease that affects us for life. Our wilderness journeys may give us a child with a developmental disability or a parent with a mental illness. The man in Luke 8:26–39, who was living among the tombs in the country of the Gerasenes and who encountered Jesus, is just one of millions of people who have suffered from mental illness, ranging from depression to schizophrenia. Our wilderness journey may cause us to fear in the middle of the night, to weep with worry, to hide ourselves in shame. Yet, we are never alone. "What are you doing here?" God asks. "How are you doing here?" God wants to know.

It is in the silence that we hear the voice of God. It is in the silence that God hears us—hears our cries, hears our worries, hears our prayers.

Our God is a God of justice. God is not on the side of those, like Jezebel and Ahab, who trample upon the poor, murdering and stealing for personal gain. Our God is a God of healing. God is on the side of those who are hiding their pain, who are afraid to come out of the cave, who fear they have lost their way. "What are you doing here, Elijah?" God asks. "What are you doing here, beloved?" God says to us all.

I work with parish nurses, and I'm often asked, "Why is parish nursing growing so rapidly?" I believe it is because parish nurses, like all of us, have lived through places of pain. As caregivers, they have responded to the call to go into the wilderness. They have left what they know—hospitals and clinics—and gone into congregations and neighborhoods to listen to others and to help others. They listen to stories of pain and loss, hope and courage. They help others understand their health conditions, and they work for healing and wholeness for all. They are nurses who responded in faith when God asked them, "What are you doing here?" Sometimes they ask themselves, "What *am* I doing here?" But more often they comment that they know they are called by God to do what they do.

Let me tell you a story about one of those parish nurses and a woman for whom she cared. The parish nurse was named Mary Ann, and she worked in another UCC church in town. I've changed the name of the parishioner—I will call her Olivia.

Olivia, an older woman, but not so very old, was recently diagnosed with cervical cancer. She told Mary Ann that she wanted two things: not to die alone, and not to die in pain. One day, when the disease had progressed to an advanced stage, Olivia fell in her house, and was moved to a nursing home. The nursing home called Mary Ann and said that Olivia was in pain, but that the hospice had not transferred her pain medications from her home to the nursing home. Olivia was moved at 3:30 P.M., but the nursing home did not call Mary Ann until 11:00 P.M. to tell her about Olivia's request for pain medication. Mary Ann called hospice and they said they could not give her pain medications because the pharmacy was closed, so Mary Ann was able to locate other pain medications for her at the nursing home. Mary Ann stayed with Olivia, holding her hand and patting her, telling her stories, and waiting until she the pain meds kicked in. Mary Ann dozed off and woke at 4:30 A.M. to find Olivia resting peacefully. She died a few minutes later. She was not alone.

Where was Mary Ann? She was in a good place, helping Olivia through the valley of the shadow of death. Where was Olivia? She was in a good place, sheltered in the loving arms of God. Where are we, today?

As the Apostle Paul wrote to the church in Rome (Rom. 3:35): "Who will separate us from the love of Christ? Will hardship, or distress, or persecution, or famine, or nakedness, or peril, or sword?" I would add, "Shall sickness, or infirmity, or the hurdle of starting an exercise program, or the stress of giving up smoking separate us from the love of Christ?"

Paul goes on to say, "As it is written: 'For your sake we face death all day long; we are considered as sheep to be slaughtered.' No, in all these things we are more than conquerors through him who loved us. For I am convinced that neither death, nor life, nor angels, nor principalities, nor things present, nor things to come, nor powers, nor height, nor depth, nor anything else in all creation, will be able to separate us from the love of God in Christ Jesus our Lord" (Rom. 8:36–39). Where are you? Wherever you are, whatever your health or condition, you are inseparable from the love of God in Christ Jesus our Lord.

Oh, by the way, we made it to the airport. I grew up on a farm, riding horses and driving tractors, so we went through the back nine. That meant we drove through the wilderness of back roads and parking lots until we got to the airport. And next week, blessed next week, we are going on vacation. We are going to a little cabin, by a little lake, back up in Canada. What are we doing there? Listening for the still, small voice of God that is within each of us, always. May you be blessed with a quiet space, too. What are *you* doing here? You are being loved by God.

May you know that the love of God is with you now and always, in every nook and cranny of your beloved and precious life. No matter what.

God bless you all. Amen and amen.

SERMON

twenty-six · **GOOD NEWS FOR LOST SHEEP**

I was sent only to the lost sheep of the house of Israel.
Matthew 15:24

Hear these words of Paul to the church at Philippi, who longed for their favorite pastor to be back with them, at a time when things were unsettled and worrisome:

> Rejoice in the Lord, always, again I will say, Rejoice. Let your gentleness be known to everyone. The Lord is near. Do not worry about anything, but in everything by prayer and supplication with thanksgiving let your requests be made known to God. And the peace of God, which surpasses all understanding, will guard your hearts and your minds in Christ Jesus. (Phil. 4:4–7)

Listen again: "The Lord is near. Do not worry about anything. The peace of God, which passes all understanding, will guard your hearts and your minds in Christ Jesus."

Comforting words, particularly in these days. Especially in this last, crazy week. Growing numbers of the poor and the not-so-poor are being evicted from their foreclosed homes. More people are showing up at food pantries. Unemployment is rising, rising, rising, and so is the number of those without health insurance.

Meanwhile, the folks at AIG who were bailed out by the government are back from a week-long retreat to California. They stayed in $500-a-night hotel rooms specially designed for travel with pampered pets. They treated themselves to $180 massages.

Paul writes to the people at Philippi like he could be writing to us today. "Beloved, whatever is true, whatever is honorable, whatever is just, whatever is pure, whatever is pleasing, whatever is commendable, if there is any excellence and if there is anything worthy of praise, think about these things. Keep on doing the things that you have learned and received and heard and seen in me, and the God of peace will be with you" (Phil. 4:8–9).

The rich getting away with what they can and the poor getting the crumbs—a new thing? Not on your life! The poor, Jesus said, we will have with us always. And apparently, also, the rich.

We just don't want to end up among the poor, and with the stock market going glub, glub, glub, it feels a little scary. No, it feels *very* scary. Especially when one factors in the unknown of health care.

I work with Deaconess Parish Nurse Ministries, whose task it is to equip registered nurses for health ministries in congregations. They provide health education and support to churches and neighborhoods. They are there to help everyone. No exceptions. It's a free service to all who need it. While many parish nurses receive a modest stipend from the church, nobody has to pay for the services of a parish nurse, just like they do not pay for the services of a clergy–person. Not so in the rest of health care, as you well know.

The rest of health care is divided into the "haves" and the "have-nots." The haves with health insurance, and the have-nots without. The have-nots suffer, delaying seeing a doctor, delay needed treatment when they do get seen, and often receive substandard care. More than eighteen thousand people each year die because they don't have health insurance.

Even those who do have health insurance face challenges. Recently, a dear family known to many on the parish nursing committee was forced to hold bake sales and have other fund raisers to raise enough money to cover the cost of a heart transplant for the young father of three, whose condition required that surgery. His mother-in-law quit her job so she could care for their children, because his wife needed to keep her job—and their health insurance. She was a chief financial officer of a large medical system, but their insurance didn't cover the full amount of their pressing needs, and the total for which they were responsible was far beyond their means. This mother was worried about feeding her family and saving her husband. By the grace of God and the generosity of her faith community and the wider community, she was able to do it.

Today's Gospel text, Matthew 15: 21–28, is about another worried mother. This mom was a Canaanite woman, not worth much in the eyes of Jesus. Her daughter was, as her mother put it, "tormented by a demon." The woman cried out, "Have mercy on me, Lord, Son of David; my daughter is tormented by a demon." But Jesus did not answer her at all.

Maybe we didn't read this right. Maybe it says, "and he had compassion on her, and he healed her." Nope. Jesus said to his disciples, "I was sent only to the lost sheep of the house of Israel." This is not in my job description, in other words. In essence, he said to the woman, "You are not part of the right group. You are not part of the right group health plan, that's for certain. You are uninsured, lady!"

But this mother didn't give up. She didn't really believe that God wouldn't want her daughter to have access to the same care that Jesus was providing to his group. She came and knelt before him. She was reduced to begging. She said, "Lord, help me."

At this point, you would have thought that Jesus would have figured it out. But he was acting like a utilization manager at this time, like God's love was finite, and needed to be rationed. He said to the woman, "It is not fair to take the children's food and throw it to the dogs." "It's not fair for those who have health insurance to subsidize the cost of paying for those who don't" would be a modern way of phrasing this.

But this was a woman who really, truly believed that God loves us. Who really, truly believed that God loves us *all*. Who really, truly believed that God's will was for healing and hope for all people in creation. Who really, truly believed that God would not abandon her. She said, "Yes, Lord, yet even the dogs eat the crumbs that fall from their masters' table." Then Jesus "got it." His eyes were open to see all people as worthy of God's love and care. His vision was expanded to encompass a mindset of abundance, not scarcity. He responded, "Woman, great is your faith! Let it be done for you as you wish." And her daughter was healed instantly.

In our Old Testament reading, in Exodus 32, the Israelites were out of Egypt, but wandering in the desert, not knowing what was coming next. They forgot the message that God loves us all and will not let us go, and so they began to get worried. They began to fret. They began to panic. They took their gold, lots of their gold, all of their gold, and sculpted it into a graven image. Aaron helped them make a new god to save them and get them through. It seems ancient, and pagan, and naive. But perhaps we, too, have been putting our faith into golden calves that are starting to crumble before our eyes. The stock market is down, the job market is down, the housing market is down, even car sales are down.

It is frightening, indeed, except that God says yes. Yes, I will love you. Yes, I will stay with you. Yes, I will lead you. Yes, I will heal you. Trust in me, says God, not in the gods you have created for yourselves. Love me, says God, with all your heart and with all your mind. Love me with all your soul and all your strength. And love, love, love your neighbor as yourself.

That love, that care, that compassion, is needed, sorely, badly needed. Forty-seven million people were uninsured in America in 2008, and that number was rising. Twenty-five million more Americans, like the family I mentioned, were underinsured, with health insurance that will not cover their medical bills. More than seventy million, or nearly one-third of all Americans under age sixty-five, were uninsured at some point during 2007–08. More than 90 percent of the uninsured were in working families. In 2008 we spent 17 percent of our gross domestic product—$2.4 trillion dollars a year—on health care. That amounted to more than $7,900 per person.[1]

In these days of personal and national fiscal belt-tightening, we must find ways to deliver the quality care we all deserve to each member of our society, and to do so in ways that saves us money—as individuals and families, and as a nation as well. Many other developed countries have health-care outcomes that are significantly higher than ours. Nearly all of those countries have achieved those outcomes at a lower cost. We are paying more—for less.

We can write letters to our elected officials, telling them that we want our state and our country to be a place where health care is available to all. We can call them on the phone. We can vote. Health care is neither a right nor a privilege. It's a commandment. Jesus said to love God with all your heart, and all your soul, and all your mind, and all your strength, and to love your neighbor as yourself. Whatever is true, whatever is honorable, whatever is just, whatever is pure, whatever is pleasing, whatever is commendable, if there is any excellence and if there is anything worthy of praise, think about these things. Keep on doing the things that you have learned and received and heard and seen in me, and the God of peace will be with you.

For God loves us. Now. And forever.
Not some of us. All of us. No crumbs.
We are welcome at God's abundant table.
And we will be fed, and blessed, and healed.
Amen.

REFLECTION

twenty-seven · **SPEAKING OF DEATH**

> *Even though I walk through the valley*
> *of the shadow of death, I fear no evil,*
> *for you are with me, your rod and your staff,*
> *they comfort me."*
>
> **Psalm 23:4 NAS**

As I write this, it is the end of summer. School will be starting again soon, and it seems strange to think about death. Signs of life are everywhere: flowers still in profusion, kids running yet once more to the pool with towels flung over their shoulders, flip-flops flying. Somehow, time has seemed suspended by heat as we have lazed by a lake, passed the day with a summer book, or just listened to the frogs. But it is perhaps at this very time, when life seems most peaceful and secure, that we should look squarely at death, at least for a time.

Over the years, I have noticed that one of the gifts parish nurses have to offer is a quiet and compassionate approach to dealing with death. Few nurses have come to parish nursing without experiencing death at work. Few have come to this stage of life without experiencing one or more deaths among close friends or family.

Theologian Dorothee Sölle's last work before her death in 2003 has been translated into English as *The Mystery of Death*. In this book, she states that while death is a limit imposed upon all, our cultures often deny the existence of limits by ignoring the reality and inevitability of death for us all.

Sölle writes, "Accepting life, admitting our limits, considering life meaningful even in its fragmentariness and brokenness, are skills we are no longer learning. The person who has learned to live only in the action mode, who finds self-justification only by doing, cannot cope with situations in which there is nothing he or she can do anymore, when limits impose themselves on us as doers."[1]

In interviews for my recent doctoral work, it was interesting to note that one of the major themes I heard repeatedly could be identified as the "ministry of presence." Parish nurses (and clergy, of course!) are willing to walk with people who are homebound and no longer doers. They are ready to sit with people whose diseases have progressed beyond cure to debilitating condition. They are prepared to remain by the bedside of those who are dying, to support and uphold the family and the dying with prayer and with care.

Death is very real. Sometimes it is a shock, sometimes a relief. Sometimes death is sudden, and other times death seems overdue. It is an important part of this blessing known as life. Who knows exactly what death precedes? Yet we know the One who precedes birth, life, and death, who goes before us, to prepare a place.

Thanks be to God for the courage of churches, where we can openly talk about death, stay close to the dying, and comfort the mourning.

REFLECTION

twenty-eight · **COMPANIONS OF COMPASSION**

> *When Jesus saw the crowds, he had compassion for them, because they were harassed and helpless, like sheep without a shepherd. Then he said to his disciples, "The harvest is plentiful, but the laborers are few, therefore ask the Lord of the harvest to send out laborers into his harvest."*
>
> Matthew 9:36-38

The word "companion" comes from the Old French word *compaignon* with the first usage noted in 1297, derived from the Latin roots *com-* ("with") and *panis* ("bread"), meaning literally "someone you break bread with." The word "compassion" also comes through Old French (1340) from the Latin roots *com–* and *pati* ("to suffer").

Certainly we suffer when our nearest and dearest are hurting—our families and friends with whom we break bread often. It is rare in health care, however, to be part of a "breaking bread" community with the people for whom you are caring. Yet that is precisely what parish nurses and health ministers do on a regular basis—they break bread with their fellow parishioners—as companions on a spiritual journey of healing and wholeness.

Parish nurses and health ministers offer hospitality (from which the word "hospital" comes, as you know). Going to the hospital can often be an anxiety-producing endeavor. There is a phalanx of personnel to encounter with name, rank, and serial number: receptionists, registration clerks, LPNs, medical technicians, radiology technicians, dietary staff, unit clerks—not even counting the RNs and the doctors who may or may not know anything about a patient other than their presenting condition. The patient is surrounded by a plethora of medical terminology, procedures, and interventions (for which we give thanks, usually!). But it is still intimidating to a patient and his or her family, and there is the concern about adverse incidents and/or infections. What a gift the presence of a parish nurse can provide fellow parishioners, as a compassionate companion on the journey of healing!

Parish nurse Gloria Wiebe asks, in her article of the same title, "Why is it so hard to talk about spirituality?"[1] Wiebe served as a compassionate companion to another RN from her parish in Toronto who was going through a painful and terrifying health crisis. She encourages us to consider whether all health-care providers should intentionally integrate care of the spirit into their professional practice. Whether or not that is possible, certainly there is great need and possibility for this care among those who break bread, suffer, and rejoice together in communities of faith in places everywhere.

REFLECTION

twenty-nine · **THE REPENTANCE THAT LEADS TO LIFE**

Then God has given even to the Gentiles the repentance that leads to life.

Acts 11:18b

When the apostle Peter was in Joppa, praying, he had a vision that the gospel of Jesus Christ was to be shared not only with the Jews but with Gentiles as well. It was a gospel of good news: transformation and new life for those who would fully embrace the message of hope. It was a new way of living—for body, mind, and spirit. All things were to be shared in common by the community of faith and they were to love and support one another—to care for their wholistic needs.

In our twenty-first-century life, our needs have been divided up. Schools and universities provide education for our minds. Clinics and hospitals provide health care for our bodies. Churches and other faith communities provide comfort and inspiration for our souls. But this artificial division of wholistic care may be harder on us than we think. It may be time for us to reclaim the vision of the early church that we can be role models for a new way of living as integrated body, mind, and spirit in community and creation.

Lloyd Rediger is a pastor in the Presbyterian Church (USA) and a pastoral counselor. He also serves as a consultant on spiritual leadership and has written several books on the topic. One of those books is a call to church leaders to turn things around and serve as role models in wholistic wellness. In *Fit to Be a Pastor: A Call to Physical, Mental, and Spiritual Fitness,* Rediger writes

What would happen if all, or nearly all, clergy in a congregation, community, denomination, nation, world, became wholly fit in body, mind, and spirit?

At first reading this sounds like a great idea but one unlikely to occur. Yet most great visions began with the inspiration of its inherent value, and wise leaders who made it happen. What if all of us who realize the vital importance of body-mind-spirit fitness decided to fan the flame of inspiration and develop a national clergy initiative?

A wave of popular consciousness-raising has already begun. Media and national leaders are citing statistics, with warnings of America's woeful lack of fitness and the enormous, largely unnecessary, costs this generates for each of us. Parishioners are becoming conscious of health and fitness issues, but many of them are unfit. Clergy are becoming conscious of health and fitness issues, but many of us are unfit. The popular expectation concerning clergy is that we will be advocates and models for the good and healthy things in life. Therefore we now have a choice: Will we help lead the fitness movement in the USA or will we be followers—or worst simply observers?[1]

Gwen Wagstrom Halaas is a physician who is active in the health ministries of the Evangelical Lutheran Church in America. She is married to a Lutheran pastor, serves as the primary care physician for a number of clergy, and has documented case studies about this aspect of her practice in her work *The Right Road: Life Choices for Clergy*. Halaas writes, "As a teacher of medical students and young physicians, I am aware of the need to lead by example and teach in a way that is practical and makes a difference."[2]

In her book, Halaas quotes data pointing to the need for a change in the lifestyles of clergy. She quotes a published study of 250 religious professionals, which found that "Protestant clergy had the highest overall work-related stress and were next to the lowest in having personal resources to copy with the occupational strain."[3] Halaas writes

This concern about the health of our church leaders coincides with a growing concern for the health of the American public. We are living in a time of "epidemics" of obesity, heart disease, diabetes, and depression. The real causes of these diseases relate to our lifestyle. We avoid activity, eat too much "fast" or processed food, work too many hours, and are isolated from our families and friends.

The fact that many of the church's leaders are overweight, inactive, depressed, and at increasing risk for heart disease and diabetes is a real concern. Taken in the context of a church in a time of declining membership, smaller and fewer congregations, older age at ordination than previously, and decreasing numbers preparing to serve congregations, this is an urgent situation.

Addressing health and wellness effectively must involve the full professional lifespan of ordained ministers and lay leaders and must be addressed in the seminaries, congregations, and administrative units of the church. We can set an example for other churches and institutions in developing faith-hardy leaders and a healthy and flourishing church. These health issues are not unique to church leaders, but are the result of American lifestyles compounded by the unique expectations and responsibilities of ministry. We will more likely be successful if we take on this initiative as families, congregations, synods, and communities.[4]

So, people of faith, what do we do? Well, many efforts are underway, and more seem to be springing forth around the country.

The National Council of Churches of the USA has a recently formed health task force that assembles representatives from Christian denominations and faith groups representing over a hundred thousand congregations. Their ground-breaking survey on health ministries in congregations provides important information for churches seeking to begin work in this area. More information about that survey can be found at www.health-ministries.org, along with a wide variety of health-related information designed for congregational use.

Some denominations, such as the Presbyterian Church (USA), the United Methodist Church, the Evangelical Lutheran Church in

America, the Lutheran Church-Missouri Synod, and the Episcopal Church, have started national health ministry programs that hold clergy leadership as central to the progress of initiatives. For example, the United Methodist Church recently announced a new Center for Health with the tagline "Fit to Lead" to address growing health concerns among United Methodist clergy and lay workers by focusing on wellness. The Center for Health will be based at the United Methodist Board of Pension and Health Benefits in Evanston, Illinois.

Speaking at a plenary session of the fourth annual National Congregational Health Ministries Conference sponsored by the United Methodist Board of Pension and Health Benefits, held in September 2008 at Lake Junaluska, North Carolina, Bishop Mike Watson, who announced the new initiative, stated,

> As a denomination, we need to empower ministries of health today so that our clergy and laity are able to continue effective ministry tomorrow and in the future. . . . We have a problem more insidious than the need for health insurance. We have an underlying health problem, and it's not getting any better. It's getting worse every day."[5]

In other places, individual clergy and lay leaders are working together to make a difference in the health of all within the congregation. There are many walking programs that are available to congregations, several of which I mention in the resource section of this book. One parish nurse, Jo Sanders, worked in partnership with her pastors, Rev. Dr. Victor Long and Rev. Deb Pollex, at the First United Methodist Church in Marion, Illinois, to offer an eight-week program, "Get My People Going!!" This wellness program included sermons, adult education, exercise, nutrition, health education, fellowship, and even a pool party. Here is what Jo said about this congregational initiative:

> We did it on eight Sunday mornings at Sunday school hour. After our preacher initially gave an amazing sermon to kick it off, we had seventy-five people come down to the altar with a commitment card to sign up. Each week an average of forty attended. We had some do it independently

because they did not want to miss their regular Sunday school classes. This worked, because we recorded the sessions each week and put them as podcasts on our church website. So, armed with the little booklet and a buddy, they could accomplish it that way too. We had forty-five minutes each week: fifteen minutes of checking in with each other and celebrating positives—motivational stuff—and then we had a speaker for thirty minutes, each week a different topic and speaker [nutrition, exercise, water, prayer and worship, Sabbath rest, community-building, and the healing power of humor]. We used our own church resources . . . the speakers were either professionals from our church, or we used friends, relatives and coworkers of members! We sent weekly e-mails and used the program materials to write things for the newsletters and bulletins. I did not spend money, really—things like pedometers, bottles of water, and handouts were donated. The church covered the expense of copying the little booklets in color, and some postage. Also each week, one of our parish nurses gave a three-minute talk about the program in both of our regular church services, so even the people who did not sign up got a little inspirational health message."[6]

Certainly, we are not yet in the promised land, but we must get going! Pastoral leadership and laity together must move forward in faith, believing that wholeness and newness of life is possible. We cannot stay here, given the challenges that are plaguing us today.

REFLECTION

thirty · THE UNDERGROUND RAILROAD OF COMPASSION

*And when was it that we saw you
a stranger and welcomed you . . . ?*

Matthew 25:38

John Hockenberry is a reporter who uses a wheelchair due to an automobile injury at age nineteen, which left him without movement or feeling in his legs. He was a student at the University of Chicago at the time of his accident, and during his rehabilitation therapy he vowed to learn how to use public transportation again. Some years later, he decided to take the subway in New York and create a radio report on wheelchair accessibility.

Hockenberry wired on a microphone to record what happened along the way. He would need to make two transfers between Brooklyn and Manhattan, which involved nearly 150 stairs. He sat down on the stairs and lifted himself up and down, while lowering and raising his wheelchair with a rope.

His attempt was an exhausting journey through crowded stations with long, filthy stairways. Most people ignored him or looked away—except for a few.

Here is what he wrote in his book *Moving Violations*: "Every white person I had encountered had ignored me or pretended that I didn't exist, while every black person who came upon me had offered to help without being asked. I looked at the tape recorder in my jacket to see if it was running. It was awfully noisy in the subway, but if any voices at all were recorded, this radio program was going to be more about race than it was about wheelchair accessi-

REFLECTION: The Underground Railroad of Compassion

bility. It was the first moment that I suspected the two were deeply related in ways I have had many occasions to think about since."[1] Accessibility. To transportation. To employment. To college. To adequate housing. To healthy food. To clean water. To appropriate health care. These are issues that people struggle with around the world and in our own backyards.

We are ministers of healing and hope. As parish nurses and clergy we need to work with others in our congregations to address issues of accessibility in the communities in which we live.

There is good information out there, starting with the Office of Minority Health and Health Disparities at the CDC (www.cdc.gov/omhd), which has health disparity information about all minorities, including persons living with disabilities. April is Minority Health Month in the United States.

Here are the words of another man who used a wheelchair: "The success or failure of any government in the final analysis must be measured by the well-being of its citizens. Nothing can be more important to a state than its public health; the state's paramount concern should be the health of its people" (Franklin Delano Roosevelt).

We are all in this together, station to station, and up those many stairs . . .

HEALING OUR INFIRMITIES
Discussion Questions

1. What are some of the ways our church offers assistance when one is experiencing an illness?

2. How do you see one's spirit affected when one is ill?

3. What are some ways in which our church could expand the ministry of compassion that it offers to those living with mental health concerns?

4. The church is one place that seems to be aware of death and its natural part of life. What does the church have to offer society, particularly given the current demographics of the aging "Baby Boomers"?

5. How is our church prepared in case of an emergency, such as a natural disaster, or a pandemic?

part six

HEALTH OF CREATION

SERMON

thirty-one · WRITE THE VISION; MAKE IT PLAIN

> Then God answered me and said:
> Write the vision; make it plain on tablets,
> so that a runner may read it.
>
> **Habakkuk 2:2**

In Nicole Mones's recent novel, *The Last Chinese Chef*, Maggie McElroy is a food writer, recently widowed. She travels to China on personal business and is given a work assignment there. Maggie is to interview Sam Liang, the American-born heir to a long line of chefs to the royal Chinese dynasties. Sam, however, has been opposed in his quest to learn the fine art of Chinese cooking by his father, also a chef. His father had suffered greatly under the Cultural Revolution of Mao Tse-Tung and vowed never to return from the United States to China.

As Maggie probes the complexities of Chinese cuisine and Sam's rising culinary star, she watches closely. Sam tells her, "A cook who is adept can create dishes that will heal the diner."

"You mean cure illness?" asks Maggie.

"Yes, but it's more than that," [Sam continues]. "People have mental and emotional layers to their problems, too. The right foods can ease the mind and heart. It's all one system."

"You cook like that?" Maggie said. "You yourself?"

"Not really. It's a specialty."

"Okay," she said, writing it down. "Healing . . . is that it?"

"One more [thing]. The most important one of all. It's community. Every meal eaten in China, whether the grandest banquet or the poorest lunch eaten by workers in an alley—all eating is shared by the group."
"That's true all over the world," Maggie protested.
"No. We don't plate. Almost all other cuisines do. Universally in the West, they plate. Think about it."[1]

Our Gospel story today (Luke 19:2–10) is of Zacchaeus, a rich tax collector in Jericho, who was in need of healing. Now, he didn't need the physical healing of a leper. He didn't need the mental healing of the man who was called "Legion." He wasn't even looking to have Jesus make him taller, despite being "short in stature." Zacchaeus was in need of an entirely different kind of restoration.

Zacchaeus, a Jew, collected taxes from fellow Jews to give the Romans in Jericho, an important commercial hub among the many countries of the Roman Empire. This would be somewhat like if the United States decided that one way to cut our taxes would be to tax citizens of countries where we had military bases. Imagine, for example, an Iraqi citizen collecting taxes from the Iraqis to send to America today.

So, Zacchaeus was probably not well liked. By anyone. In addition, he admits in this story to defrauding some people even beyond what the Romans expected them to pay. This guy was in real need of healing.

Jesus looked right up at him in that sycamore tree and said

"Zacchaeus, hurry and come down, for I must stay at your house today." So he hurried down and was happy to welcome him. All who saw it began to grumble and said, "Jesus has gone to be the guest of one who is a sinner." Zacchaeus stood there and said to the Lord, "Look, half of my possessions, Lord, I will give to the poor; and if I have defrauded anyone of anything, I will pay back four times as much." Then Jesus said to [Zacchaeus], "Today salvation has come to this house, because he too is a child of Abraham and Sarah. For I came to seek out and to save the lost." (Luke 19:5b–10)

The Greek word for "salvation" used in this text is the word *soterion*, which means "keep from harm, rescue, heal, or liberate." Surely Zacchaeus was rescued, liberated, *and* healed.

Jesus healed the mind of Zacchaeus, certainly. He took away the nagging worry at the back of his mind that would never go away. Jesus healed the spirit of Zacchaeus, when he believed in the authenticity of his repentance. He healed the social health of Zacchaeus when he said that he would stay at his house. He pulled Zacchaeus back into community. And he brought healing to the world when he said to the crowd, "Today salvation has come to this house, since Zacchaeus is also a child of Abraham and Sarah. For I came to seek and to save the lost."

Nowadays when we talk of healing, we often mean individual health. Wholistic health, to be sure, but just one person's health at a time. Body, mind, and spirit.

But Jesus went beyond the concept of body, mind, and spirit and connected the person back into community. And not only that, he connected communities to the fullness of God's creation.

It is what the Christ wants for us all.

In our Western world, where our food is plated and our houses are mostly single family homes, we hardly know the neighbors on our street, let alone our neighbors in South America, Asia, or the Middle East.

Come, Lord Jesus, be our guest.

And let this food, this house, this community, this world be blessed.

"Write the vision; make it plain on tablets, so that a runner may read it. For there is still a vision for the appointed time; it speaks of the end, and does not lie. If it seems to tarry, wait for it; it will surely come, it will not delay. Look at the proud! . . . They gather all nations for themselves, and collect all people as their own" (Hab. 2:2–3).

We are in need of healing. Some of us need healing for our bodies, some for our minds, some for our spirits. And we all need healing for our communities and our world. There is much to be done, but we stand on the shoulders of the saints who have gone before us. We are surrounded by a cloud of witnesses. We are surrounded by our grandparents who believed this to be a good land, in a good earth. We are surrounded by our parents who believed in us and gave us the legacy of life. We are surrounded by our families, our neighbors, and all the saints who fill this glorious creation.

Sam Liang's Chinese grandfather, the one who had cooked for the emperor, had written,

> In this humble book I have tried to give the facts about the cuisine of the Chinese imperial palace. It was a place of tragic beauty. Of everything I learned there, one thing stands out. Food was always to be shared. When my master sent out his untouched dishes from the huge imperial repasts to the families of the princes and the chief bureaucrats, he would send them only as complete meals for eight people in stacked laquerwear. Never any other way. Always for eight. The high point of every meal was never the food itself; he taught us, but always the act of sharing it.[2]

God has called all the saints to share—to share our food, to share our gifts, to share our vision for healing and wholeness in the world. Healing and wholeness of body, mind, spirit, community, and creation. God has invited all to the table, not as one person, but as one body, the body of Christ. Now and forevermore. Amen.

SERMON

thirty-two · **THE EARTH IS SATISFIED**

You make springs gush forth in the valleys; they flow between the hills, giving drink to every wild animal; the wild asses quench their thirst. By the streams the birds of the air have their habitation; they sing among the branches. From your lofty abode you water the mountains; the earth is satisfied with the fruit of your work.

Psalm 104:10–13

I would like to take a moment to tell you about the amazing work of Alvyne Rethemeyer, who was the first director of parish nursing at Deaconess Parish Nurse Ministries in St. Louis, from 1995 through 2007.

Alvyne, in her ministry of healing, had much in common with Jesus, the Great Nurse. For starters, there's the thing about their names. The angel said, "He shall be called Emmanuel," so they called him Jesus. Alvyne's parents said, "She shall be called Alvyne," so everyone calls her Alvihn, or Alvin, or Alvina.

Jesus said things that were true and hard to hear. For example, he said, "It is easier for a camel to go through the eye of a needle than for a rich person to receive the realm of God." Alvyne also says true and hard things, such as, "You're not as young as you used to be, you know."

Then there's the thing about Jesus walking on water. Alvyne may not be able to do this, but for a number of years she taught a water walking class at the Y. So, you decide for yourself.

Like Jesus, Alvyne, and *all* ministers of health, teach others how to heal. Parish nurses and ministers teach others to affirm their value to God, no matter what their physical condition. Christ would have us honor and care for our bodies, the temple of God's spirit. Christ would have us build community, welcome the stranger, care for the little ones. Christ would have us care for the earth—God's earth—ours to use as faithful and caring stewards while we are here.

Now, you may think it very strange that the text chosen for this sermon would be an obscure passage from Psalms. There are so many wonderful stories of healing in the Bible! Healing the lepers, curing the demon-possessed, putting mud on the eyes of a blind man. But the vision of healing and wholeness that the church is to be about is more than "here's mud in your eye!" It's about having meaningful work and peaceful rest. It's about living in community with all God's creation. That's a tall order for any community.

But it's a typical order for the church. Congregations around the country are out there, helping senior citizens in their homes and starting summer school programs for kids. They are starting housing programs and teaching parenting classes. Clergy, parish nurses, and others are working together to provide care and healing for body, mind, spirit, community, and creation. Parish nurses are helping groups with dementia to reminisce and those healing from trauma to trust. They lead exercise groups, weight loss groups, parenting support groups, grief support groups. They promote healthy nutrition, help people find jobs, take abused women to shelters. The church prays with people, cries with people, hopes with people.

Jesus was a carpenter, and he cared about the whole house! He didn't just care about the roof—that triangle on top of body, mind, and spirit (see diagram). He also drew the connections down into the community and into all of creation. We can't be healthy if we have no friends. We can't be whole if creation is groaning, and global climate change is just one indication that creation certainly is groaning! Jesus wanted the whole house to be strong!

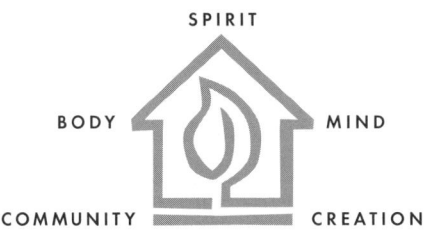

God's healing is for us—for our bodies, our minds, and our spirits. But it is also for our communities, and for our creation. And we are partners in that healing care. It makes sense that we care deeply about whether or not our water is clean. It makes sense that we care deeply about whether or not our food is safe. It makes sense that we care deeply about whether or not our air is clean. It seems like a huge issue. But the huge nature of the issue only is that the care of creation has become a political issue. Our Scriptures remind us that care of creation is also a theological issue.

What can we do this day to affect the environment positively? The choices we make about heating and cooling our church facilities and our homes will affect the environment. The choices we make about maintaining these buildings will affect the environment. Our choices regarding food, clothing, cars—in fact, around most of the things that we have and use, affect the environment.

We give thanks for this marvelous creation—for the springs that gush forth, the animals that fill the forest, and all good gifts. And we pray for wisdom as we seek to bring healing to this community, and into all your precious world.

REFLECTION

thirty-three · WHERE HAS ALL THE OXYGEN GONE?

> *Then God formed a person from the dust of the ground,
> and breathed into the being's nostrils the breath of life; and the person
> became a living being. And God planted a garden . . .*
>
> **Genesis 2:7–8a**

Not far from the little place my husband and I own in the Ozarks is a beautiful tree-covered mountain, once a majestic volcano, formed one and a half billion years ago. At the end of the road is a sawmill, to which trucks bring logs and from which trucks take wood to be made into magazines. Recently, the owner of the mountain property began to clear-cut slopes and a rapidly spreading baldness is appearing.

On trips from the city, my kids love tapes and have mercifully graduated from Raffi and Elmo to such classic singers as Peter, Paul, and Mary. As I listened to "Puff, the Magic Dragon" again, I thought of another folk classic—"Where Have All the Flowers Gone?" A war protest song, it translates well into today's environmental situation—"Where have all the forests gone? Gone to paper, every one. When will they ever learn? When will they ever learn?"

When will *we* ever learn? Is the environment something that parish nurses should worry about? Joyce Rupp, in her book *The Cosmic Dance* writes,

> When I used to hear facts about the termination of species, global warming, and destruction of rich farm lands and rain forests, I felt badly but did not think it affected me. I

had absorbed the cultural lie that I was not connected to the land, creatures, sea, or air. . . . Every day I am offered the tremendous gift of sipping from the mystery of life, tasting the exquisite beauty in what the universe offers me from the vast cup of the cosmos. And in the midst of this beauty, I am also invited to hear the groan of suffering that arises from our bleeding and wounded planet.[1]

She states that an acre of trees produces oxygen for eighteen people.[2] According to the U.S. Census Bureau, the world's population is nearly seven billion. We need a lot of trees, if we want to breathe easy.

It does cost a few cents more for tissue made from recycled paper. Seventh Generation, a company that produces environmentally safe household products, claims that if every home in the United States replaced just one small box of tissues with recycled ones, eighty-seven thousand trees would be saved, as well as landfill space equal to 330 garbage truck loads and thirty-one million gallons of water.

How much can parish nurses do? They can do what they can! We here in our office use recycled paper for the copier and in our restrooms. We've switched to phosphate-free dish soap in our kitchen. How is protecting the environment part of your wholistic health ministry? What more can we all do?

May we work together to preserve the blessing of sweet forests and air for our children and our children's children.

REFLECTION

thirty-four · **PRAYING FOR THE HEALTH OF THE WORLD**

*The earth is God's
and all that is in it, the world,
and those who live in it.*

Psalm 24:1a

Edwina Gately is a Catholic laywoman who cares deeply about the health of the world. Originally from England, Edwina worked in the 1960s as a missionary in Uganda, where she founded a girls' school that became the largest and most successful in the area. In the 1980s, she went to seminary in Chicago and then started Genesis House in that city as a mission to women in prostitution. At age fifty, she adopted an infant, and now her work is raising her child and writing. Edwina has written a number of books, including *Whispers*, about prayer and following God's call within your life.

Edwina writes:

> In times of crisis and suffering, think about how comforting it is to have someone we trust praying for us, focusing their thoughts on our problem and bringing those thoughts to God in silence. Somehow, in a way we cannot understand, that makes a difference. We are all connected. We affect one another whether we feel it or not. We are comforted and grateful when somebody is thinking of us or praying for us. So when contemplatives pray for the world, the world may not understand what they are doing, but something deeply spiritual does happen. And, of course,

the contemplative prayer of any of us, for whatever period of time, affects the world too. We have not even begun to understand the effect that we can have on each other and on society when we pray, when we tap into the divine source within us and we project the healing grace from that source onto the brokenness of an individual or the brokenness of our world.[1]

As I write these final chapters of this book, it is a troubling and worrisome time in the world. The stock market has plunged in ways that resemble the start of the Great Depression. Job losses are mounting, and millions are losing their homes. The number of the uninsured is rising. Global climate change remains a challenge to us all.

There is much to do for the healing of our communities, our nation, and our world. Yet we are not alone.

Be assured that you are in our prayers. Please keep us in yours.

REFLECTION

thirty-five · **HEALING CHRISTMAS**

> *Look, the virgin shall conceive and bear a son,*
> *and they shall name him Emmanuel,*
> *which means, "God is with us.*
>
> **Matthew 1:23**

In his book *The Sacred Santa*, Dell deChant argues that our culture is deeply religious, but following a religion far different from Judaism, Christianity, or Islam. He calls this new religion "Consumer Economics." Under this religious system, people seek to find meaning and purpose in the acquisition, consumption, and disposal of consumer goods. Christmas can be a time when we are particularly challenged by the lure of consumption and drawn away from that which brings true life.

Howard Thurman, a beloved pastor and at the time of his death dean emeritus of Marsh Chapel at Boston University, wrote, "Hope is the mood of Christmas: the raw materials are a newborn babe, a family, and work. Life keeps coming on, keeps seeking to fulfill itself, keeps affirming the possibility of hope."[1]

What does this these mean for congregations? Well, the holidays will be upon us again shortly. They are a wonderful, yet challenging time for those who promote the health of faith communities. Can we tone down the overindulgence and wild expectations of Christmas? Can we set a simple mood that brings healing and hope? Can we bring healing to Christmas?

Just think of the issues that may arise in a congregation around the holidays:

Food: The holidays are a hard time to stay on a diet, yet doing so is important, particularly for those who are on special diets due to chronic illness.

Drink: Alcohol is related to a number of health concerns and adds to the severity of violence when abuse is present in a family system.

Loneliness: Isolation is often a contributing factor to health problems. The holidays are a hard time to be alone, especially when one is grieving the loss of a loved one.

Shame: Families are pressured to shower gifts on their families and friends, often in ways far beyond their means. Credit debt is soaring.

So what can parish nurses and health ministers do to promote wholeness within this culture? Here are some ideas:

Stay connected to your parishioners. Listen to them share stories that may help you understand where you, the pastor, or another congregational member may be of help.

Use newsletter articles and bulletin boards to promote healthy eating, drinking, and spending during the holidays.

Suggest an alternative Christmas fair at church, where homemade items may be sold at a reasonable cost, or to which not-for-profit organizations selling fair trade items such as those available through "Ten Thousand Villages" could be invited.[2]

The church needs to proclaim that we are not able to eat, drink, or buy our way to happiness at Christmas or any other time of the year. When we worship the one true God, the holidays remain about love, connection, and wholeness! Blessings to you all.

REFLECTION

thirty-six · **GOD'S EARTH, OUR INHERITANCE**

> *The earth is God's and all that is in it,*
> *the world, and those who live in it:*
> *for God has founded it on the seas,*
> *and established it on the rivers.*
>
> **Psalm 24:1**

In *Gift from the Sea*, Anne Morrow Lindbergh travels to an island off the coast of Maine, near where she had spent time as a child, to recover, somewhat, from the deep wounds of terrible loss—the kidnapping and death of her eldest son, Charles Lindbergh Jr. The sea, and the gifts it brought her, became a source of great healing for Anne. In her book *Dakota*, Kathleen Norris finds spiritual resources within herself and in relation to her faith community through her observations of the sacred in nature. And who has not been blessed by the descriptions of nature in the deeply spiritual writings of Annie Dillard?

We are one with nature, and yet we often live so "at two" with it. We depend on the creation around us to provide our food and the raw materials for all our possessions—our homes, our clothing, the very ground we walk on, and the air we breathe. We cannot live without depending upon the bounty of nature, yet we take it for granted, and we seem to be causing it harm. The growing numbers of animals joining the ranks of endangered species is great cause for alarm. The causes for global climate change might still be debated, but it is clear that the climate is, indeed, changing. We are in challenging economic times, and when economic challenges in the 1930s were coupled with severe, long-term drought, we had a very great depression indeed.

The earth may be God's, and the fullness thereof, but it is our inheritance, and we must tend it well for our children. The Iroquois believed that decisions about the earth should be made with the next seven generations in mind. How seldom we have done so!

Dorothee Sölle, in *To Work and to Love: A Theology of Creation*, writes,

> The earth is sacred. Ten years ago I was not so conscious of the sacredness of the earth. It is when we are confronted with the utter threat to that which we love that we rediscover the wellsprings of our love and realize our interdependency anew. The conspiracy to undo creation—or even part of it—in a "winnable nuclear" war reignites our awareness of the sacramentality of the earth, or the earth's nondisposability (*Unverfügbarkeit*), to borrow Martin Heidegger's term for existence. The earth is not disposable. Some of its resources are not renewable. We did not create the earth, but we are its stewards.[1]

We are no longer able to ignore the growing plight of our earth, given the tremendous increase in the world's population and the tremendous increase in our consumption of its resources. Most middle-class families in America now have a car for each driver, a TV for most rooms in the house, several computers, and a small army of household appliances. Few American cities have public transportation that is adequate for daily use by most of its citizens, and almost none are entirely pedestrian-friendly (let alone hospitable to the person using a walker or a wheelchair).

We consume much larger portions of food at meals than our families did fifty years ago, and we eat more meat, which requires more water and feed for livestock. Water is growing scarce in some of our major cities, and brownouts are becoming more common.

Does the church have any role at all to play in the health of creation? Or should we focus our health ministries solely on physical health of our bodies—that which we can more easily control? After all, Reinhold Niebuhr wrote, "God, give us grace to accept with serenity the things that cannot be changed, courage to change the things that should be changed, and the wisdom to distinguish the one from the other." Maybe we should be wise enough to know that improving the health of our world is simply beyond us. Or is that just fatalism? Surely there is something that we can do to make a difference!

Mark I. Wallace, in *Finding God in the Singing River: Christianity, Spirit, Nature,* writes, "The environmental crisis is a spiritual crisis because the continued degradation of the earth threatens the fundamental interconnections that bind human beings to one another and to all other forms of life."[2] If this is, indeed, a spiritual crisis, then the church must be at the center of this debate.

Indeed, it has been at the center of this debate for centuries. Willis Jenkins, in *Ecologies of Grace: Environmental Ethics and Christian Theology,* points to the theological writings of Thomas Aquinas, Karl Barth, Walter Brueggeman, Emil Brunner, Martin Buber, John Cobb, Sallie McFague, Thomas Merton, Jürgen Moltmann, Origen, Rosemary Radford Reuther, and Pierre Teilhard de Chardin (among others).[3] Theologians have been discussing this topic for centuries. For some faith traditions, including Anabaptists, such as the Mennonites, Amish, and Hutterites, their careful use of resources have been central to their religious practices for centuries as well.

One of the more well-known resources from this latter tradition is the book *Living More With Less*[4] by Doris Janzen Longacre, a Mennonite author who also wrote the *More-With-Less Cookbook*, which is subtitled, "Suggestions by Mennonites on how to eat better and consume less of the world's limited food resources."[5] These suggestions for living and eating are drawn from the worldwide experience of Mennonites who had lived in a variety of developing countries as well as across the United States.

What is the legacy that each of our congregations will leave related to care of God's creation, our earthly inheritance, and that of our children, to the seventh generation, and, we pray, beyond?

HEALTH OF CREATION
Discussion Questions

1. In what ways does our congregation reach out to others around the world?

2. How could we expand our global connections?

3. What could our congregation do to further support the environment through our buildings?

4. What could our congregation do to further support the environment through our grounds?

5. Where in our church structure could we build accountability for efforts toward wholeness of creation?

Notes

PREFACE AND ACKNOWLEDGEMENTS

1. From the Introduction in "Silence Kills: Speaking Out and Saving Lives" in *Creative Non-Fiction*, Issue 33 (Pittsburgh: Creative Nonfiction Foundation), 2007.

CHAPTER ONE: MOVED BY AUTO RICKSHAW

1. Dorothy Clarke Wilson, *Ten Fingers for God* (New York: McGraw-Hill, 1965), vii–viii.

CHAPTER TWO: NO JOY FOR YOU?!

1. Based on an ancient antiphon from *Advent Vespers*, translated by John Mason Neale, 1851, and others, public domain.

CHAPTER THREE: KIDNEY STONES AND OTHER LEARNING EXPERIENCES

1. Wilson, *Ten Fingers for God*, 145.

CHAPTER FOUR: MYSTICS, VISIONARIES, AND HEALERS

1. "I Would Be True," hymn text by Howard Arnold Walter, 1906, public domain.

CHAPTER FIVE: MINISTRY LOVES COMPANY

1. John T. Galloway, *Ministry Loves Company* (Louisville: Westminster John Knox Press, 2003), 3.

CHAPTER SEVEN: IF RELIGION WAS A THING THAT MONEY COULD BUY

1. 2000 U.S. Census Bureau statistics.
2. Kaiser Commission on Medicaid and the Uninsured, a policy brief of the Henry J. Kaiser Family Foundation, September 2008, http://www.kff.org /medicaid/7815.cfm, accessed October 6, 2008. Statistics change with time, and readers are urged to revisit the websites cited in this book for updated health-care data.
3. "Who Are the Uninsured?" Robert Wood Johnson Foundation report, compiled from September 2001.
4. 2006 data from the Agency for Healthcare Research and Quality, part of the U.S. Department of Health and Human Services, as quoted by the Coalition for Affordable Healthcare Coverage in "Meet America's Uninsured," www.cahc.net/meet.html, accessed June 4, 2009.
5. Ibid.

6. U.S. data from the Centers for Medicare and Medicaid Services (CMS), reported in the National Coalition on Health Care document "Health Insurance Costs," http://www.nchc.org/facts/cost.shtml, accessed June 4, 2009.

7. Forty-two percent of U.S. medical schools closed or merged within two decades of the Flexner report, 12 percent as a direct result of the report, according to Mark D. Hiatt, M.D., M.S., M.B.A., and Christopher Stockton, M.S.M, "The Impact of the Flexner Report on the Fate of Medical Schools in North America after 1909," *Journal of American Physicians and Surgeons* 8/2 (summer 2003): 37ff., downloadable in pdf format at www.jpands.org/vol8no2/hiattext.pdf, accessed June 4, 2009.

8. "Large Raise for Executive at Hospital Stirs Criticism," *New York Times* April 3, 2004.

9. An HMO president's salary was $369,000 on average in 1996, according to Pam Pohly's Netguide. Ms. Pohly was a hospital administrator and CEO for Tenet Healthcare from 1987 to 1990.

CHAPTER EIGHT: REWRITING YOUR FUTURE

1. Isabel Allende, *My Invented Country: A Nostalgic Journey through Chile* (San Francisco: HarperCollins, 2003), 87–88.

CHAPTER NINE: PRAYING FOR HEALTH CARE

1. S. Brink, "Coverage, in Pieces," *Los Angeles Times*, April 3, 2006.

2. S. M. Asch et al., "Who Is at Greatest Risk for Receiving Poor Quality Health Care?" *New England Journal of Medicine* 354/11 (2006): 1147–56.

3. L. Sanders, "Medicine's Progress, One Setback at a Time," *New York Times Magazine*, March 16, 2003.

4. H. Benson et al., "Study of the Therapeutic Effects of Intercessory Prayer (STEP) in Cardiac Bypass Patients." *American Heart Journal*, 151/4 (2006): 934–42.

5. N. Kristof, "Hazardous to Your Health," *New York Times*, April 11, 2006.

6. C. Schoen et al., "Taking the Pulse of Health Care Systems," *Health Affairs* Web exclusive Nov. 3, 2005, international survey, http://www.commonwealthfund.org/Content/Publications/In-the-Literature/2005/Nov/Taking-the-Pulse-of-Health-Care-Systems—Experiences-of-Patients-with-Health-Problems-in-Six-Countri.aspx, accessed June 4, 2009.

CHAPTER TEN: HEALTH CARE FOR AN ARM AND A LEG

1. Reported by Ceci Connolly and Kendra Marr in "As Budgets Tighten, More People Decide Medical Care Can Wait," *Washington Post*, October 16, 2008.

2. Ibid.

3. Patricia Gleich, partner, Lifespan Enrichment Consulting Services and former associate for National Health Ministries, PC (USA), e-mail correspondence January 20, 2007, quoted with permission. Gleich can be reached at myhealthyagain@gmail.com. See also Kaiser Daily Health Policy Report," January 19, 2007, http://www.kaisernetwork.org/daily_reports/rep_index.cfm?hint=3&DR_ID=42366, accessed October 16, 2008.

4. U.S. data from the Centers for Medicare and Medicaid Services (CMS), reported in the National Coalition on Health Care document "Health Insurance Costs," http://www.nchc.org/facts/cost.shtml, accessed June 4, 2009.

5. Ibid.

CHAPTER ELEVEN: DOWNSTAIRS ON A FIRST-NAME BASIS

1. Epigram at the beginning of chapter 6, "Pudd'nhead Wilson's Calendar," *Pudd'nhead Wilson and Other Tales* (first serialized in *The Century Magazine*, 1893–94; edition quoted from Oxford: Oxford University Press, 1992), 34.

2. "Westberg as a Patient" in *Granger Westberg Verbatim* (St. Louis: International Parish Nurse Resource Center, 2003), 55.

2. Peter S. Bernstein, MD, MPH, "Care of Patients in Groups: The New Model of Healthcare," http://www.medscape.com/viewarticle/529462?src=mp, accessed May 19, 2006.

CHAPTER TWELVE: THE HARDEST WORDS

1. David Maxfield, Joseph Grenny, Ron McMillan, Kerry Patterson, and Al Switzler, "Silence Kills: The Seven Crucial Conversations in Healthcare," report on the AACN website, www.aacn.org/WD/Practice/Docs/PublicPolicy/SilenceKillsExecSum.pdf, accessed October 6, 2008.

2. Ibid.

CHAPTER FOURTEEN: AND THEIR EYES WERE OPENED

1. Carl Sandburg, *Abraham Lincoln: The Prairie Years* (New York: Harcourt Brace & Company, 1926), 77, as quoted in Richard A. Hasler, *Surprises Around the Bend: 50 Adventurous Walkers*, (Minneapolis: Augsburg Fortress, 2008), 73.

2. Philip B. Kunhart Jr., Philip B. Kunhart III, and Peter W. Kunhart, *Lincoln: An Illustrated Biography* (New York: Knopf, 1992), 321, as quoted in Hasler, *Surprises*, 73.

3. Hasler, *Surprises*, 74.

4. Carl Sandburg, *Abraham Lincoln: The War Years* (New York: Harcourt, Brace & Company, 1939), 177–79, as quoted in Hasler, *Surprises*, 74.

5. As printed in *Mark Twain's Speeches* (New York: Harper & Brothers, 1910), 425–34, accessed June 5, 2009 at http://etext.virginia.edu/railton/onstage/70bday.html.

6. Joyce Rupp, *Walk in a Relaxed Manner: Life Lessons from the Camino*. (Maryknoll, N.Y.: Orbis Books, 2005), 54.
7. Ibid., 77.

CHAPTER SIXTEEN: THEREFORE, CHOOSE LIFE

1. Gary Gunderson and Larry Pray, *The Leading Causes of Life* (Memphis: Center for Excellence in Faith and Health, Methodist LeBonheur Healthcare, 2006), 169–70.
2. Viktor Frankl, *Man's Search for Meaning* (New York: Simon & Schuster, 1963), 157.
3. From chapter 1 of Reinhold Niebuhr's *The Irony of American History* (Chicago: University of Chicago Press, 1952), http://www.press.uchicago.edu/Misc/Chicago/583983.html, accessed September 24, 2008.

CHAPTER EIGHTEEN: WE DO NOT LIVE BY STRESS ALONE

1. Rob Stein, "Baby Boomers Appear to Be Less Healthy Than Parents," *Washington Post*, Friday, April 20, 2007.
2. Ibid.

CHAPTER NINETEEN: SUFFER THE CHILDREN

1. Leslie T. Chang, "Gilded Age, Gilded Cage," *National Geographic*, May 2008, http://ngm.nationalgeographic.com/2008/05/china/middle-class/leslie-chang-text, accessed June 9, 2008.
2. Norimitsu Onishi. "For English Studies, Koreans Say Goodbye to Dad," *New York Times*, June 8, 2008.
3. "Substance Abuse Prevalence among Teens Is High," *Science Daily*, http://www.sciencedaily.com/releases/2007/11/071105164456.htm, accessed June 9, 2008. Study published in *Archives of Pediatric & Adolescent Medicine* 161/11 (2007): 1035–41.
4. "About Family Day," http://casafamilyday.org/familyday/about-family-day/, accessed June 4, 2009.

CHAPTER TWENTY: THE WISDOM OF ELDERS

1. Personal correspondence between Nancy and her parish nurse, Ellen. Quoted with permission.

CHAPTER TWENTY-ONE: LORD, HELP US!

1. For more information, visit the website of the National Institute on Disability and Rehabilitation Research at http://www.ed.gov/about/offices/list/osers/nidrr/index.html.
2. National Institute of Mental Health (part of the National Institutes of Health), "What are the Autism Spectrum Disorders?" http://www.nimh.nih.gov/health/publications/autism/what-are-the-autism-spectrum-disorders.shtml, accessed June 4, 2009.

3. Karen Siff Exkorn, *The Autism Sourcebook* (New York: Harper Collins, 2005), xiv.

4. Howard J. Clinebell Jr., *The Mental Health Ministry of the Local Church* (Nashville: Abingdon Press, 1965), 15.

CHAPTER TWENTY-TWO: IDENTIFIED: FLYING TOILETS

1. Celia W. Dugger, "Toilets Underused to Fight Disease, U.N. Study Finds," *New York Times*, November 10, 2006.

CHAPTER TWENTY-SIX: GOOD NEW FOR LOST SHEEP

1. National Coalition on Healthcare, http://www.nchc.org/facts/cost.shtml, accessed April 3, 2009.

CHAPTER TWENTY-SEVEN: SPEAKING OF DEATH

1. Dorothee Sölle, *The Mystery of Death* (Minneapolis: Augsburg Fortress, 2007), 15.

CHAPTER TWENTY-EIGHT: COMPANIONS OF COMPASSION

1. Gloria Wiebe, "Why is it so hard to talk about spirituality?" http://www.articlearchives.com/medicine-health/medical-treatments-procedures/1885464-1.html, reprinted from the spring 2008 newsletter of the Parish Nurse Interest Group (PNIG) of the Registered Nurses Association of Ontario (RNAO).

CHAPTER TWENTY-NINE: THE REPENTANCE THAT LEADS TO LIFE

1. G. Lloyd Rediger, *Fit to Be a Pastor: A Call to Physical, Mental, and Spiritual Fitness* (Louisville: Westminster John Knox Press, 2000), 167.

2. Gwen Wagstrom Halaas, *The Right Road: Life Choices for Clergy* (Minneapolis: Augsburg Fortress, 2004), ix.

3. C. A. Rayburn et al, "Men, Women, and Religion: Stress within Leadership Roles," *Journal of Clinical Psychology* 42/3 (1986): 540–46, as cited in Halaas, *The Right Road*, 1–2.

4. Halaas, *The Right Road*, 4.

5. Deborah White, "New Center for Health Focuses on Clergy, Lay Workers," UMC Featured News and Stories, September 28, 2008, http://www.umc.org/site/apps/nlnet/content3.aspx?c=lwL4KnN1LtH&b=2433457&ct=6016435, accessed October 15, 2008.

6. E-mail correspondence with J. Sanders, used with permission. See also the website of the First United Methodist Church in Marion, Ill., www.marionfirst.org, to access the initial sermon, "Fearfully and Wonderfully Made," delivered June 8, 2008. Click on Sermons on the left side of the home page. Then click on any of the podcasts to hear the speakers. For more information on the "Get My People Going!!" program, contact the International Parish Nurse Resource Center at www.parishnurses.org or call 314-918-2559.

CHAPTER THIRTY: THE UNDERGROUND RAILROAD OF COMPASSION

1. John Hockenberry, *Moving Violations: War Zones, Wheelchairs, and Declarations of Independence* (New York: Hyperion, 1995), 308.

CHAPTER THIRTY-ONE: WRITE THE VISION; MAKE IT PLAIN

1. Nicole Mones, *The Last Chinese Chef* (Boston: Houghton Mifflin, 2007), 37.
2. Ibid., 266.

CHAPTER THIRTY-THREE: WHERE HAS ALL THE OXYGEN GONE?

1. Joyce Rupp, *The Cosmic Dance: An Invitation to Experience Our Oneness* (Maryknoll, N.Y.: Orbis Books, 2002), 18–19.
2. Ibid., 18.

CHAPTER THIRTY-FOUR: PRAYING FOR THE HEALTH OF THE WORLD

1. Edwina Gately, *Whispers: Conversations with Edwina Gateley* (Trabucco Canyon, Calif.: Source Books, 2000), 100–101.

CHAPTER THIRTY-FIVE: HEALING CHRISTMAS

1. Howard Thurman, *The Mood of Christmas* (New York: Harper & Row, 1973), 20.
2. Ten Thousand Villages is a program of the Mennonite Central Committee. More information is available on their website at www.tenthousandvillages.com, where you can locate a partner store near you, or contact them at Ten Thousand Villages, 704 Main Street, PO Box 500, Akron, PA 17501-0500 or toll-free at 877-883-8341.

CHAPTER THIRTY-SIX: GOD'S EARTH, OUR INHERITANCE

1. Dorothee Sölle, *To Work and to Love: A Theology of Creation* (Philadelphia: Fortress Press, 1984), 3.
2. Mark I. Wallace, *Finding God in the Singing River: Christianity, Spirit, Nature* (Minneapolis: Augsburg Fortress, 2005), 28.
3. Willis Jenkins, *Ecologies of Grace: Environmental Ethics and Christian Theology*x (New York: Oxford University Press, 2008).
4. Doris Janzen Longacre, *Living More With Less* (Scottdale, Pa.: Herald Press, 1980), and its companion *Living More With Less Study/ Action Guide*, written by Delores Histand Friesen (Scottdale, Pa.: Herald Press, 1981).
5. *More-With-Less Cookbook* (Scottdale, Pa.: Herald Press, 1976).

Resources

PART ONE: CALLED TO HEALTH MINISTRY

These organizations have a plethora of information on health ministry:

International Parish Nurse Resource Center—www.parishnurses.org
475 E. Lockwood Avenue, St. Louis, MO 63119
314-918-2559

Health Ministries Association—www.hmassoc.org
Box 529, Queen Creek, AZ 85242
480-358-4709

Also, be sure to visit these websites for more information on health ministry:

Australian Faith Community Nurses Association—www.afcna.org.au

Australian Parish Nurse Resource Center—www.apnrc.org

Canadian Association for Parish Nursing Ministry—www.capnm.ca

Ecumenical Health Care Ministry Council (Bahamas)—
www.geocities.com/healthcareministry/ecumenical.htm

InterChurch Health Ministries (ICHM) in Canada—www.ichm.on.ca

New Zealand Faith Community Nurses Association—
www.faithnursing.co.nz

Northwest Parish Nurse Ministries—www.npnm.org

Nurses Christian Fellowship—ncf-jcn.org/index.html

Parish Nursing Ministries UK—www.parishnursing.co.uk

Presbyterian Church (USA) National Health Ministries—
www.pcusa.org/health/usa/parishnursing/primer.htm

National Council of Churches Survey—
www.councilofchurches.org/healthsurvey/

National Episcopal Health Ministries—
www.episcopalhealthministries.org

Spiritual Care Collaborative—www.spiritualcarecollaborative.org

United Church of Christ Parish Nurse Network—
www.ucc.org/justice/health/ucc-community-nurses

United Methodist Parish Nursing—www.gbgm-umc.org/parishnursing

PART TWO: ACCESS TO HEALTH CARE

These organizations have a great deal of current information on access to health care, and there are many others as well.

- Families USA—www.familiesusa.org
- Henry J. Kaiser Family Foundation—www.kff.org
- Robert Wood Johnson Foundation—www.rwjf.org
- US. Census—www.census.gov (click on "Health Insurance")

PART THREE: HEALTHY LIFESTYLES

You can find more information than you can possibly use all over the web. Good websites can be found through the National Institutes of Health (www.healthfinder.gov), the Mayo Clinic (www.mayoclinic.com), and WebMD (www.webmd.com).

Also, contact your local hospitals, local health department, and local medical schools for more information. They often offer free speakers and sometimes free health screenings for your groups.

PART FOUR: HEALTHY FAMILIES

Here is an outstanding website for children's health information, sponsored by Nemours, the largest children's healthcare organization in the US: www.nemours.org. Also good are Kidshealth at www.kidshealth.org, and the part of the Medline Plus website designed for children's health, www.nlm.nih.gov/medlineplus/childrenshealth.html.

Family Day: A Day to Eat Together™ is a wellness initiative of the National Center on Addiction and Substance Abuse (CASA) at Columbia University, 633 Third Avenue, 19th Floor, New York, NY 10017-6706 (212-841-5200). More information can be found at www.casafamilyday.org, where free downloadable materials are available.

The National Alliance on Mental Illness (NAMI) is a great organization that assists congregations that want to help individuals and families dealing with mental illness. Website: www.nami.org; address: Colonial Place Three, 2107 Wilson Blvd., Suite 300, Arlington, VA 22201-3042; and toll-free phone number: 800-950-NAMI.

Finally, the AARP has good resources about health care. Go to the website at www.aarp.org, and click on "Health."

PART FIVE: HEALING OUR INFIRMITIES

See parts three and four above.

PART SIX: HEALTH OF CREATION

There are growing numbers of organizations working on sustaining the health of the planet. One good place to start is the Sierra Club (www.sierraclub.org), which is likely to have a chapter near you. Also, contact your denomination to join national efforts in this arena.

Bibliography

Clinebell, Howard J. *The Mental Health Ministry of the Local Church.* Nashville: Abingdon Press, 1965.

deChant, Dell. *The Sacred Santa: Religious Dimensions of Consumer Culture.* Cleveland: Pilgrim Press, 2002.

Gunderson, Gary, and Larry Pray. *The Leading Causes of Life.* Memphis: Center for Excellence in Faith and Health, Methodist LeBonheur Healthcare, 2006.

Halaas, Gwen Wagstrom. *The Right Road: Life Choices for Clergy.* Minneapolis: Augsburg Fortress, 2004.

Hasler, Richard A. *Surprises Around the Bend: 50 Adventurous Walkers.* Minneapolis: Augsburg Fortress, 2008.

Jenkins, Willis. *Ecologies of Grace: Environmental Ethics and Christian Theology.* New York: Oxford University Press, 2008.

Oswald, Roy. *Clergy Self-Care: Finding a Balance for Effective Ministry.* Washington, D.C.: Alban Institute, 1991.

Rediger, G. Lloyd. *Fit to Be a Pastor: A Call to Physical, Mental, and Spiritual Fitness.* Louisville: Westminster John Knox Press, 2000.

Rupp, Joyce. *The Cosmic Dance: An Invitation to Experience Our Oneness.* Maryknoll, N.Y.: Orbis Books, 2002.

———. *Walk in a Relaxed Manner: Life Lessons from the Camino.* Maryknoll, N.Y.: Orbis Books, 2005.

Sölle, Dorothee. *Death by Bread Alone: Texts and Reflections on Religious Experience.* Philadelphia: Fortress Press, 1978.

———. *The Mystery of Death.* (Minneapolis: Augsburg Fortress, 2007).

———. *To Work and to Love: A Theology of Creation.* Philadelphia: Fortress Press, 1984.

Thurman, Howard. *The Mood of Christmas.* New York: Harper & Row, 1973. Rpt, Richmond, Ind.: Friends United Press, 1985.

Wallace, Mark I. *Finding God in the Singing River: Christianity, Spirit, Nature.* Minneapolis: Augsburg Fortress, 2005.